Manual for Urine Therapy Teachers & Therapists

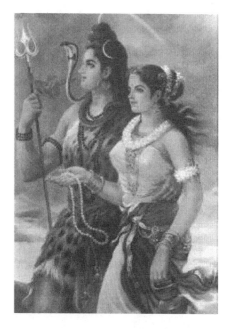

Brother Sage
foreword by Dr. David Jubb

Manual for Urine Therapy Teachers & Therapists

How to deepen your knowledge of Urine Therapy, Masterfully teach and guide other people's UT process And be a successful Urine Therapist

Copyright © 2020 by Brother Sage
1st printing: December 2020; 2nd edition: January 2024

Cover design by Brother Sage
www.brothersage.com

Created for print and ebook by Lampas Books
www.lampasbooks.com

ISBN (print) **979-88-772321-6-7**
An electronic copy of this book is also available
on Amazon.com

Footnote codes (*resources) (†references)

Contents

Introduction   13

Chapter 1: History of Shivambhu   17

Chapter 2: Why Shivambhu matters for humanity?   25

Chapter 3: How faith or trust play a role in UT   27

Chapter 4: Orin is everyone's perfect elixir.
How does Shivambhu work?   31

Chapter 5: Research and Clinical Studies on Urine
Therapy   52

Chapter 6: The whole body/mind connection way
to supercharge AUT effectiveness through
optimum diet, attitude, emotions, and self-love
practices   60

Chapter 7: UT protocols. Introducing saturation dosing,
sip looping, and new protocols discovered between
2019-2020   64

Chapter 8: Offering suggestions without prescribing or
diagnosing   160

Chapter 9: General treatment suggestions   164

Chapter 10: Designing UT protocols and wellness
practices for a client to bring radiant health   173

Chapter 11: Clearing the mind of all negative associations,
beliefs or ideas about UT, including suggestions,
theories, and myths taught to you, especially
by the medical industry   176

Chapter 12: Surveying a client   190

Chapter 13: Preparing for a UT session   193

Chapter 14: Looking into an Orin Therapy session   197

Chapter 15: Presenting your UT service professionally   214

Chapter 16: Presenting your UT service professionally
to the media. Some proven promos that will bring
greater interest in your work   221

Chapter 17: To charge or not to charge for your services   228

Chapter 18: What the experts say about AUT   233

Chapter 19: Shivambhu Master Teachers and superstars   254
Chapter 20: The Future of the Shivambhu movement and
      Urine Therapy   259
Chapter 21: Humor as a therapeutic adjunct to AUT does
      make a difference   267
Chapter 22: Shivambhu a 501C3 non-profit organization
      Shivambhu Hut, the First alternative Social Media
      platform focused just on UT   272
Last word from Author   285
About the Author   287

Foreword

Brother Sage is at it again with another masterpiece. Read and learn the secret to immortality and a long life. Look between the covers of this book and discover a little-known truth today. Get in on the cutting edge now, and anticipate this new work on one of the most important topics that you could possibly explore: Urine Therapy. It is here to stay.

—Dr. David Jubb*

Prayer

May this manual attract an abundance of inspired urine therapy enthusiasts who are ready to become Urine Therapy teachers or therapists.

May all readers learn the true meaning and value that AUT (auto urine therapy) holds for them in their lives.

Learn how to master AUT, how to share it freely, and how to guide students in their progress along their personal AUT Journey.

Discipline and enthusiasm is required on this *sacred water path* secret to success. Develop a unique way of working with clients that transforms them, you, and everyone.

May *your water of personal aliveness* be a constant source of wisdom, regeneration, inspiration, consciousness evolution, and well being.

Somewhere in this manual, you will discover why being a teacher of one of the oldest and highly respected professions in the world, Urine (Orin) Therapy, called to you.

Ultra filtered, activated, distilled, golden blood plasma water, aka Orin (a term made popular by Andrew Norton Webber), needs your voice to spread this important message.

Welcome to the water family.

Breathe.

Sharing Orin Therapy experiences, teachings, suggestions, and insights with others and posting online *does matter.* This helps everyone. Sharing this message everywhere you can support and helps Shivambhu devotees and the movement reach millions more and continue to make a difference.

Dedication

This manual is dedicated to devoted and outspoken UT teachers, advocates, and enthusiasts worldwide who are sharing AUT in their work both locally and internationally.

We honor and recognize some of the renowned and outstanding individuals who are still making a difference in the lives of their many clients (whether these teachers are alive or not). Some have maintained a UT practice for over 50 years.

Visit the Resources section of this book for a list of prominent and noteworthy UT teachers. Reach out to them for advice, suggestions, or to acknowledge them.

Thank you, Shiva, for nourishing us with every precious drop of this amazing water.

Bless you for being among the growing number of Orin Therapy enthusiasts, educators, and therapists. Your courage, openness, devotion and willingness to share your AUT wisdom to anyone who is ready to listen and perhaps get started, makes you a Shivambhu superhero.

> "Without question, I drink my water when delivered, or I save every drop for practicing the protocols and storing it to allow it to evolve."
>
> —George Johnson, USA

> "I absolutely drink my pee, doesn't everyone?"
>
> —Indira Bhatt Gupta, India

The regenerative (Shakti) power of Shivambhu awakens an innate knowledge (Brahman) of the original genetic blueprint and memory of your body and soul. A body's infinite intelligence demonstrates its love for you by continually producing ultra-filtered, activated, and evolving nutrients in the most perfect blend and timing for you.

As such, only the healthiest substances will remain after Orin returns its travels back into the bloodstream—and ultimately to produce another trillion cells.

"You may think that when it comes to alternative health therapies you've heard it all. But there is one natural therapy you've probably never heard of—even though its one of the most powerful, most researched, and most medically proven natural cures ever discovered."

—Martha Christy

Urine Therapy: it may save your life!

"For almost the entire course of the 20th century, unknown to the public, doctors and medical researchers have been proving in both laboratory and clinical testing that our own urine is an enormous source of vital nutrients, vitamins, hormones, enzymes, stem cells and critical antibodies that cannot be duplicated or derived from any other source.

They use urine for healing cancer, heart disease, allergies, autoimmune diseases, diabetes, asthma, infertility, infections, wounds, and on and on— yet we're taught that urine is a toxic waste product. This discrepancy between the medical truth and the public information regarding urine is ludicrous and, as the news releases you've just read demonstrate, can mean the difference between life and death to you and to your loved ones."

—Martha Christy

Introduction

In light of recent global events of the year 2020, this book will shed some light on human self-health care.

Concerned about the uncertainty or any health risk of taking vaccines as a prevention or cure for infections or contamination by a virus or the effects of other human-made dangers we are facing today?

Instead of waiting for a vaccine to appear to save you or debating if taking a vaccine will put your health at risk, there is a natural self-healing alternative you can take today.

What can we learn from over 5,000 years of healings and recoveries that are being recorded daily by tens of millions of people in 50 "known" countries?

Historic and modern Ayurvedic practitioners, yogis, Judaic/Christian/Greek/India/Roman/European traditions, naturopaths, natural health and wellness professionals, along with courageous talk show hosts are presenting UT to their clients, viewers, networks, and the world.

This approach to free self-health care is becoming increasingly known either by word of mouth or from those who source their news and information from social media and alternative sources—not from the mainstream media.

The ancient remedy, practice, and lifestyle, as presented in this manual, has proven itself as a panacea (cure-all) by the many today who are practicing AUT.

Like many natural remedies, our perfect medicine is known by the medical system and the media. These controlled systems are instructed to ignore UT, however; they spread negative propaganda or simply push their services, drugs, and/or agendas.

The exploding Shivambhu movement is being fueled by growing number of social media groups and platforms comprising some 500,000 members (various websites, YouTube channels, and personal contacts who are sharing their experiences). They are lending incredible support and encouragement to others who are on the Shivambhu journey.

There is one water with one strong voice made of the voices of millions that is spreading the message of a lifetime: *Shivambhu*.

Remind your students to keep an open mind so they can learn, understand, and accept this incredible gift of life. The subject of this manual requires a simple willingness to accept and understand a new idea and the possibility that it may be an answer to millions of prayers.

As we study and really get to know the truth about AUT, which is that same life-giving water in which we spent 9 months of the primary stages of our lives growing, we will also gain the knowledge and skills of a well-trained UT teacher or therapist.

Breathe

Are you ready to meet the mind of an AUT prospect and possibly a client or student?

Are you serious about moving into one of the oldest known professions, which has been around much longer than prostitution?

One's confidence to teach others about

AUT will come naturally by simply practicing the protocols daily. From self-healing and involvement with your practice, UT soon becomes a lifestyle and a way of being.

Never underestimate the power of the worldwide water family for their incredible support, comfort, and friendship. They are a safe community that allows you talk about Orin and be yourself.

Being a "product of the product" comes naturally to those who practice AUT every day. You are building a solid foundation of health to last a lifetime and perhaps beyond.

This consistency not only gives you optimal health, but it will also inspire you to serve everyone who finds his or her way to you and Orin Therapy.

This creates a lasting bond of trust and a sense of relief to your clients and students.

The information in this manual has been masterfully written for your Orin Therapy career to begin. Your confidence in understanding the experiences as you work along with the manual to grow your AUT practice will make the difference in the lives of countless people who will be looking to you as a teacher to guide them through their current health and life challenge(s).

Living water that matters!
Tell the world.

You felt the pull or calling to take this path. This says that you are ready to develop the skills and understanding of Shivambhu or AUT.

Instead of using the word *urine* in this manual, popular words or terms for urine from various cultures and traditions will be used as a replacement.

For the sake of this manual, you will be acquainted with some of the many alternative terms for Orin. The word *urine* is from the Latin *urina*, which is from the variant of the Proto-Indo-European root *awer*, meaning "to moisten" of "to flow."

The word *piss* is an onomatopoetic term for urine and has been used since before the 14th century. (*Onomatopoetic* refers to the formation or use of words, such as *buzz* or *murmur*, that imitate the sounds associated with the objects or actions which they refer.)

The word *piss* came into use to describe the sound that orin made while peeing.

There are many names used to honor and define Orin from multiple cultures or traditions. Here are just a few to wet your whistle:

Shivambhu is the traditional Hindu spelling of the word. Shivambhu: *bhu* means water. It means water of Shiva or blood of the Lord, Amaroli, Amrita, water of auspiciousness, Nectar of Immortality, golden blood plasma water, water of personal aliveness, intuitive water, Ito (Nigeria), Lodha Cola (term made popular by Dr. Rakshak Mal Lodha of India), "U" Juice (from Stampana Osenotse of Botswana), Orina (Spanish speaking countries), Water of Life, Orin Juice (the new OJ) or Nectar of Immortality.

Whether a client has a mild or severe health challenge, your confidence, patience, compassion, and trust in the process is all you need to guide clients on their UT Journey.

Whether you are new to AUT, an experienced Orin enthusiast, or you just bought this manual to do more research of our out of mere curiosity, you will gain fuller knowledge and insight into how daily use of the Water of Life creates the health, happiness, and vitality you deserve.

This manual will answer all the questions that your clients may have. This manual addresses concerns, considerations, or beliefs about drinking pee delicately.

Sometimes the simplest answer to questions about the effectiveness and health benefits of orin is the best answer.

You are standing in the position where it is your responsibility to give the reassurance to the uncertain mind of the client that together this challenge will be resolved.

Here's my favorite answer to the question, "Can Orin Therapy heal this condition or that condition?"

This following reply makes it really clear that you are not a trained medical professional and not qualified to diagnose or write prescriptions.

"I don't know about that, all I do know is that when I drink my wee or rub it on my body, I feel better."

You are a teacher or therapist and a guide for the client's education and progress toward balance and well-being.

You will be getting very close to your clients, and there will be discussions about inner wellness (their deepest held beliefs about themselves).

It is perfect that you are doing this work or you would not be reading this book.

A "spiritual presence" will be with you and felt by you, without even mentioning it.

Being clear on your knowledge about AUT will move you to share it openly, confidently, and honestly. When clients feel safe with you, they tend to open up and admit that they are either ready to learn about AUT or that they have been practicing Orin Therapy.

As you become known for your work with AUT, more people will be confessing that they have been drinking pee, that they were too embarrassed and kept it a secret, or that they are relieved to come out of the water closet and tell someone.

It is now safe and on purpose for me to tell people about AUT.

It's all in the mind.

Chapter 1
History of Shivambhu

The use of orin (urine) for the healing all ailments is traced back over 5,000 years to a god or deity in the Hindu tradition, known as *Shiva*. Shiva represents goodness, benevolence, and protection.

Shiva is associated with time, particularly as the creator and destroyer of all things seen and unseen. He brings creation to all of life as well as destruction of all illusions.

Shiva, the lord of the Universe, along with his divine partner, Parvati (goddess of fertility, love, beauty, marriage, children, devotion, divine strength, and power) is remembered for bringing Orin Therapy (Shivambhu) to humanity.

FYI: Their elephant son, Ganesha, is acknowledged for removing of obstacles by many people.

The ancient Damar Tantra scriptures teach a 9-year course on how to use Orin Therapy to achieve perfect health, longevity, and ultimately physical immortality.

That's why the idea of drinking your own water is respectfully known as *Shivambhu*, which literally means the water of Shiva or blood of the Lord.

Devotees refer to orin as the "water of auspiciousness" because its benefits have been documented with tens of thousands of testimonials from people across earth that have healed themselves using their own water.

Traditional or indigenous healers in India, Africa, German, Australia/New Zealand, and 45 other countries have been practicing and teaching AUT for millennium.

To understand the obvious, doctors trained in the Western or allopathic tradition of medicine, tend to see Orin therapy as hooey.

The worldwide water family feels otherwise

Despite the theory by the modern medical industry, that Orin is a waste product, it is actually *ultra-filtered golden blood plasma water*. Lifesaving blood plasma is what first responders give to their patients while driving them in the ambulance on the way to the hospital.

It is this same golden blood plasma that the kidneys receive from the liver and process though a system consisting of millions of filtration chambers known as the *nephrons*.

The nephrons distill (the word "distilled" comes from the root "dis" meaning to make opposite. *Dis-tilled water is really activated water)* the smallest particles taken from the blood plasma transporting it to the bladder. Here, the orin sits waiting for that pressure to signal for you to do something with it— which is to pee.

One of the honored names for urine include *orin* (a term made famous by *Andrew Norton Webber). *Orin is Aquaman's birth name.* Aquaman learns that his birth name was Orin and that he and his enemy Ocean Master share the same father, "an ancient Atlantean wizard" named Atlan (Source: Wikipedia).

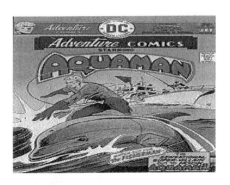

Modern Medical and Scientific Aspects of Auto Urine Therapy

Over the years, AUT has proven to be an effective tool for self healing. Most Orin teachers, some of whom have been practicing UT for decades, never sought an explanation for why or how it works: their own experiences were sufficient proof.

However, there has been an increasing interest in the search for a valid scientific explanation. Why? Because UT teachers believe it is important for UT to be acknowledged as an accepted method of healthcare treatment.

A doctor should be well-informed about the effects of AUT so their staff and client's families can make a sound decision about starting UT and how it will benefit them from its use.

Let this be the day that *the narrowminded and contolled medical system wakes up,* having studied and accepted the documentation and scientific research and publicly acknowledge that *Orin really is our perfect and free medicine.*

Another reason for this growing interest is that a number of mainstream doctors have also had positive experiences with UT, which is reason enough for them to investigate how and why it works.

This is not a recent development. In the 1930s, for example, the German pediatrician Martin Krebs successfully treated many patients with UT and subsequently published the results. As a physician he was convinced that UT was an effective method of treatment but he also realized that other *doctors would not readily accept this fact since it conflicted with the scientific dogma that formed the foundation of their profession.*

In order to be able to acknowledge UT as an effective method of treatment, a number of the world's medical doctors are building an interest in how it works. Discovering how it actually works, however, will take work. Random, double-blind, crossover research could be useful but is difficult to execute.

Research has already been conducted within the medical system into the composition of orin and its 1,000 components. The researchers Free and Free published a report that *pointed out that these are only the most significant substances, and that orin contains over 3,000 identified components.*

Several substances found in orin have proven valuable for use as medication, cosmetics, and agriculture, some of which are been processed and used.

A number of hypotheses have, however, been suggested that can serve as the basis for further scientific research.

According to Dr. Bartnett, applying orin therapy, using self-produced orin (*or pee from anyone*) can be considered as an extension of the methods of Jenner and Pasteur.

An important task of the immune system is to rid the human body of diseased or unusable substances that have developed, which has lead up to an illness. When the substances in orin reach healthy tissue, the serum or blood becomes stronger, the activity of leukocytes (white blood cells) increases, and the patient recovers.

This phenomenon is known as *self-vaccination and can be seen as Mother Nature's methods of healing an illness without any external intervention.*

UT can also be seen as a form of self-vaccination: certain bodily substances that have been removed from the body, some of which may have been produced as a result of illness, are reintroduced into the body in small amounts. These substances are re-absorbed into the blood through either the intestines or the skin. According to this hypothesis, the immune system is then given the chance to respond appropriately.

The doctors Remington, Merlin, and Lennon have demonstrated that a particular part of orinprotein is able to eliminate pathogens. This discovery supports the assumption that UT can be used to treat or prevent illnesses.

In the early 19th century, Dr. Charles Duncan conducted research into therapies with self-produced substances, including UT. He demonstrated that patients suffering from gonorrhoeic urethritis (infection of the urinary tube as a result of the venereal disease gonorrhoea) produce their own medication in the form of their own water.

AUT was applied here by placing a drop of a patient's orin directly on the tongue, in order to stimulate the body's natural powers. This method has a strong healing effect at every stage of an illness. When orin is applied at an early stage it causes the gonorrhoea to disappear and be healed much sooner.

The results of Dr. William D. Linscott's research suggest that AUT strengthens and stimulates the immune system, in particular with regard to the T-cells. The T-cell population of several patients who initially displayed a low T-cell count had increased after a UT treatment.

Chapter 2
Why Shivambhu matters for humanity?

In the 21st century, Shivambhu addresses the needs and health challenges of humanity. Shivambhu illuminates the overuse of resources, energy, finances and personnel for health care for now and for future generations.

The world is facing water and food shortages along with a major physical and psychological health crisis. Shivambhu is here to bring a unified solution to all personal concerns and worldly conditions.

Mass distribution of this manual will allow the awareness, education, and resources of this practice to deliver this self-health care information to the many concerned and desperate beings everywhere.

Since our water *is* the perfect medicine, complete with every known nutrient required by the body for optimum health, many consider Orin *as the mother of all super foods.*

Not only does orin meet and exceed our nutritional needs, it also has been known to satisfy hydration or thirst.

As an answer to both hunger and thirst, Orin may be just what the world needs as a source of food and water for thriving.

Auto Urine Therapy (AUT) can awaken self-love and well-being in everyone.

"Zindabad"
"Long Live Shivambhu!"

—Indira Bhatt Gupta

Chapter 3
How faith or trust plays
a role in UT

Shri Santabalji considered Orin Therapy to be the boon of nature and a blessing by God for humanity. He describes human orin as a divine and most powerful medicine. God has shown us this sure cure of all diseases. The truly wise person considers Orin as the best of all cures. Its prowess is indestructible.

All of the many opinions about AUT are worth considering with an open mind. It can be seen in all religions and ancient Indian sects, including the Jains and the Buddhists who have considered the Orin cure to be a sure cure.

Even the researchers are also slowly but unreservedly approving the sterling qualities of UT. All these opinions and verdicts are good eye-openers.

Has it occurred to you that Shivambhu is

your water of personal aliveness, well-being, and possible road to physical immortality?

Without questions, concerns, or fears about getting better, you know that Shivambhu is healing you or has healed you by now.

Orin is the perfect elixir arriving in the most perfect timing when you need it.

Faith clears obstructions, inflammation, toxins and pathogens, as these are being cleansed and released permanently from the body.

Faith reminds you that you will never have to buy or use supplements or medications because it's all in the water.

Faith in Shivambhu will guide you to choose living foods, lighter foods, less food or no food without resistance or conflict.

Faith in Shivambhu clears the mind so creativity, imagination, and curiosity will re-awaken.

Of course, not everyone is ready for this leap of faith, which is to begin drinking *pee*. Instead of obsessing over taste and smell, *orin* is a sample of what is flowing through your veins and any repulsive *orin* is a motivation to improve the internal conditions, *rather than an excuse for not using Orin Therapy*.

Moment by moment it is Faith (also known as *trust*) that is steadying and balancing you.

Faith is guiding and carrying you while you are navigating the mind though its endless stream of ideas.

100% *no money back* GUARANTEE

Trust in your own living water, along with a daily practice utilizing a variety of UT protocols and you will achieve perfect health, well-being, abundance, and overwhelming feelings of gratitude for life.

Our holy water purifies, cleanses, restores, and regenerates every area of life. Healing yourself or reclaiming your body occurs while the mind and spirit are being realigned; thanks to the related nutrients found in orin.

Shivambhu devotees report a richness and greater quality of life. Their clear minds blended with a calm relaxation and joy brings them home to their natural way of being.

Thanks to you, Shivambhu, I am now at peace and am enjoying all the beauty, blessings and bounty in this moment.

Faith is sending me one client at a time that is eager to return to a superior quality of life.

My faith is increasing, so are my client's faith and their daily AUT practice. The results are becoming exhilarating and transformational for us both.

Above all things, have faith in the Presence or the Light in us all.

Now take the Shivambhu message to the world that is seeking answers to their health matters.

Chapter 4
Orin is everyone's perfect elixir. How does Shivambhu work?

A Nutrient-rich Powerhouse

In 1975, one of the founders of Miles Laboratories, Dr. A. H. Free, published his book *Urinalysis in Clinical Laboratory Practice*, in which he remarked that not only is orin a sterile body compound (purer than distilled water), but that it is now recognized that orin contains thousands of compounds.

From among the orin constituents mentioned in Dr. Free's treatise, check out this *list of nutrients that will knock your socks off.*

Adrenaline, Alanine, Albumin, Allantoin, Antibodies, Amino acids, Arginine, Ascorbic acid, Bicarbonate, Biotin, Calcium, Carbohydrates, Chloride, Choline, Cortisone, Creatinine, Cystine, DHEA, Dopamine, Enzymes, Epinephrine, Estrogen, Folic acid, Glucose, Glutamic acid, Glycine, Hormones, Inositol, Insulin, Iodine, Iron, Leucine, Lysine, Magnesium, Manganese, Melatonin, Methionine, Nitrogen, Ornithane, Oxytocin, Pantothenic acid, Phenylalaline, Phosphorus, Potassium, Progesterone, Proteins, Riboflavin, Selenium, Serotonin, Stem Cells, Sulfur, Testosterone, Thiamine, Tryptophan, Tyrosine, Urea, Vasopressin, Vitamins A, B6, B12, C, D, E, K & Zinc.

In addition to the above substances Orin is an excellent "biofeedback" machine. It contains the broken-down products of the metabolism of each of our trillions of cell. These particles carry *up-to-date information* on the exact status of the health of each individual cell at any given moment of time.

It also contains other products manufactured by the body to counteract any ailment.

Orin is a perfect "telltale" and excellent diagnostic agent. Thus, for instance, Vitamin A is not normally excreted in the orin but in patients with cancer and tuberculosis large quantities of Vitamin A can be detected.

The composition of orin changes from season to season and, in fact, moment to moment. Lack of sleep, poor food choices, and unhealthy eating habits, grief, and happy moments each influence the composition of orin.

If we had sophisticated instruments to detect each and every particle present in orin, we would get a perfect scan of the functioning of all cells present in the body (which are particular to a specific moment when examined) and perhaps know the complex role is performed by the body to restore health.

The functions of the main substances in orin are described below:

The presence of antigens and antibodies in orin strengthens the immune system when it is reintroduced into the body. The reintroduction of small amounts of bacteria or parasites found in orin may stimulate the production of IgA (a virus inhibiting substance that prevents microorganisms from becoming embedded in the mucous).

IgA is found in mucous and in excretions

of the body, and therefore also in orin. UT increases the production of IgA, which explains why orin has a positive effect on infections of the urinary passages, and the kidneys while other treatments offer little relief.

Urea is the major component found in orin and is the end product of protein metabolism. It dissolves fats and other body secretions and is finally released into the orin. As a strong antibacterial agent, orin specifically prevents the growth of the tubercle bacillus and other pathogens.

Uric acid is similar in action to urea and has strong antibacterial properties. In addition it helps to control cancer-causing substances.

If nitrates present in the orin, come in contact with the skin or sweat, they will react with the acid producing nitrous oxide, *which is antibacterial.*

Minerals from orin can be very easily absorbed when reingested and become more efficient compared to minerals derived from food. Orin contains different kinds of useful mineral compounds than those derived from fruits and vegetables.

All the minerals in the biological substances were once absorbed from food, processed, and then eliminated as surplus.

Orin becomes turbid (cloudy or hazzy) when left alone for a while. This is because when enzymes in orin change urea into ammonia, orin becomes unstable and strongly alkaline. Therefore, evolving orin looks cloudy.

Orin with higher ammonia content when applied to the skin plays an important role in beautifying it.

Minerals in orin purify and activate body tissues, which were not purified by the blood. In addition, they mobilize the toxins while facilitating their excretion. Minerals help rebuild tissues.

Cortisone found in orin counteracts inflammatory conditions, allergies and other skin diseases.

Melatonin (maintains your wake-sleep cycle) and serotonin (a chemical needed for the nerve cells and brain to function) present in the morning orin have a stress reducing effect. It boosts the immune system, support glandular functions, inhibits cancer, and reduces heart disease.

It is known to have a rejuvenating effect. This explains why many who practice UT prefer to drink the first collected orin of the day.

Urokinase detected in orin dissolves

blood clots, helps cure heart disease, and improves blood circulation.

Epithelium Growth Factor (EGF) helps repair and regenerate damaged tissues and skin cells.

Colony Stimulating Factor (CSF) is necessary for cell division and multiplication.

Growth Hormone (GH) shows different bioactive effects, such as promotion of protein production, cartilage growth and fat decomposition.

Erythropoietin, a hormone secreted by the kidneys, promotes production of red blood cells in response to falling levels of oxygen in the tissues.

Gonadotropin hormones, which have a stimulating effect on the gonads, normalises the menstrual cycle and sperm production.

Kallikrein releases kallidin which expands peripheral veins and reduces blood pressure.

Trypsin Inhibitor is effective for prevention and healing of mucosal tumors (neoplasma).

Allantoin (which is also found in beets, comfrey, aloe vera, and wheat sprouts) heals wounds by repairing tissue and tumours and reverses aging.

Adrenocorticotrophic Hormone (ACTH)

stimulates adrenal cortex to make cortisone.

Thyrotrophin (TSH) stimulates thyroid gland and controls energy (ATP) turnover in the body.

Leutenising Hormone (LH) stimulates sex hormone production.

Follice Stimulating Hormone (FSH) supports menstrual cycle and pregnancy.

Parathyroid Hormone regulates calcium metabolism.

Anti-cancer substances like antianeoplaston H-11, beta-indol-acetic directin, 3-menthy glyoxal differ from chemotherapeutic drugs that kill or injure all kinds of cancer cells.

They strongly prevent the multiplication of carcinogenic cells and help return them to normal.

Stories have been told of individuals who have both lived and died by being trapped in places without food and water for days. *Those who survived did so because they drank their own orin; those who perished did not.* The ones who died probably could not overcome the misinformed thoughts that orin is a waste product of the body. *It is not.*

Orin is a *living water* that the body urinates that contains elements not needed at the time.

Such claims about the power of Shivambhu come easy with inhabitants of oriental East, where orin has long ben viewed as the body's own pharmacy or medicine chest. In the West, UT is currently in vogue with the more adventuresome followers of yoga and with others who are seeking alternative ways to prolong life and maintain radiant health.

Some individuals came to UT as an extension of their adopted philosophies (Hindu, Taoist, Native American, Maori, etc.), while others came out of sheer desperation—seeking the "urine cure" purely on its on reputed merits, with little or no interest in exotic Eastern or indigenous belief systems.

While some urine drinkers use it only as an occassional tonic—to correct temporary imbalances or diseases—there are actually many others who down a glassful of orin every day or all day (as in the case of looping or orin fasting) as part of their daily health regimen. Just how widespread is this practice?

Hard figures for most nations are, understandably not available (yet). However, in June 2001, Chinese news feeds reported that more than 3 million Chinese people drink their own orin to stay healthier. That's 3 million cups of pee a day, every day—just in mainland China alone.

Despite what you may have been led to believe about orin, pharmaceutical companies gross billions of dollars from the sale of drugs made from orin constituents. Research is happening every day in labs attempting to isolate specific elements of orin so they can create new drugs and patent the substances.

For instance, Pergonal and Metrodin are fertility drugs being made from the *orin of postmenopausal nuns*. 1992 sales of this drug are reported at $855 million while it costs a patient $1400 a month to consume. **Nuns, Woah!**

Urokinase, an orin ingredient, is used in drug form and sold as a miracle blood clot dissolver for unblocking coronary arteries. Therapeutic-grade Urea, *medically proven* to be one of the best moisturizers in the world, is packaged in expensive creams and lotions.

Take the M out of Murine eye drops and what do you have? Yep. It's made from carbamide—another name for synthetic urea.

Since this manual serves as a training book for teachers, UT testimonials will not be included. There are links to several websites with testimonials in the *Resources section* near the end of the book. Follow or share the links to find testimonials to healing illnesses with Shivambhu. Perhaps there are several testimonials that you may be searching for yourself or someone else.

Chris Bociek ▸ Urine Therapy: THE REAL UNIVERSAL REMEDY
6h ·

I'm a Rock dude....I grew up playing in a Thrash Metal band...i was the drummer\singer...now I play trippy rock. I have been sick my whole life with different diseases....I have had ITP, I have Crohn's....i have symptoms of everything under the sun...i even went blind in one eye. Then one day on a medication website i was trying (that covered my whole body in rashes and bumps) i ran into Brother Sage, and he told me about UT....that dude changed my life by reaching out to me......I've Partied my ass off, done a ton of booze and drugs obviously that goes with the lifestyle...lot's of mental problems, a messed up family with tons of sickness and mental illness....the list is too long....UT BROUGHT ME BACK!!!! ANYONE who is thinking of trying this DO IT!@! It's the single most helpful thing I've ever done for my health I'm 46 and i've been sick pretty much since the day i was born....Aged rubs on the neck and torso completely take away my mental illness, and help my Crohn's....internally i drink a bit of fresh, and I take a half ounce aged mixed with coconut water here and there....LIFE CHANGING....I have just finished my album...played every instrument myself on it and sang it....best accomplishment of

... my life, and I don't think I could have done it without this....STOP READING ABOUT IT AND SAVE YOURSELF...just keep experimenting until you find what is comfortable to YOU.. remember to try and do the rubdowns and drink...rubdowns with aged are SO awesome. After it ages for about a month and a bit it stops smelling bad too....put it on neck torso, and armpits for lymph, let it sit for an hour or two and take a shower...for best results do the rubdown then sit in the sun....you might even get high off it like a mild mushroom buzz...and you get a huge hike in your spiritual awareness and abilities. BEST THING EVER!!! Cheers to Brother Sage for reaching out.

👍 Like   💬 Comment

👍 6

Ramana Shiu
I am learning from you too
2h · Like · Reply

Rakshak Mal Lodha
Best wishes
Brother Sage is professor of Urine Therapy

Since clients come to you for guidance; they trust you and rely on your suggestions or advice for their improvement and return to well-being.

When asked how Orin Therapy works, *try this reply*. Understanding the unique qualities of Orin Therapy and how it works is to understand its nature, its nutritional components, substances, significance, and supernatural power.

Some approach this question in various directions based on their understanding of healing and especially self-healing.

I have spent 4 decades as a wellness practitioner, teaching nutrition as an answer to health concerns, but it was not until 1994 that I was given direction to begin practicing Shivambhu directly from Shiva.

After 26 years of practicing Shivambhu saturation protocols, I credit my good health, energy, good attitude, and vitality to the practice and use of using this perfect intuitive water every day.

Orin is the best and last supplement that I will never buy

Many "water brothers and sisters" are being called by Shivambhu and simply know and trust that it works.

The way to know for sure that Shivambhu can be an answer to your health and wellness takes discipline or commitment. Not only will you see results soon, you will be able to live a long and healthy quality of life by maintaining a continual daily practice.

How does orin affect attitude, emotions, and behavior? Thanks to the presence of various hormones and nutrients, drinking or topically applying orin balances and improves one's attitude while restoring better brain health.

Orin delivers vital nutrients to the brain, as it repairs important functions and raises alkaline pH, and it reduces tension and inflammation as it removes toxins and pathogens.

Benefits from UT include: feeling good in your body, better confidence (better sense of self), concentration, mental peace, improved memory, clarity, and creativity.

Thanks to orin, with nutrients such as serotonin, melatonin, oxytocin, magnesium, B vitamins and DHEA, people report feeling calm, patient, and safe.

With the absence of chemicals that cause addictions, many have gained their freedom from these self-destructive habits within a week of drinking pee.

This newfound confidence has been inspiring many UT enthusiasts to radically change and improve their food choices (some call a diet), even move toward living foods or a fruitarian lifestyle.

Shivambhu, like breathing, is a miracle

Q: Are there any exceptions to who can benefit from UT?

A: No. AUT can be practiced by anybody whether they are young, old, babies, sick, or healthy without any expenditure and with a little basic knowledge.

It does not produce any side effects, after effects or ill effects, which are generally unavoidable with the use of medicines or surgery. AUT treatments are fast, inexpensive (free), harmless, safe and simple to administer for any chronic or acute illness without the help from any doctor or medical professional.

Shivambhu devotees are healthy people who rely on UT to remain healthy. Whereas, a sick person can be free of their challenges very promptly. UT is self evident, self-contained and reliable source of the water of life.

Q: Can pets be treated with orin therapy?

A: Many of the research tests on orin recycling have proven it works well with animals. Veterinarians have successfully used Orin Therapy at clinics as a treatment by administering orin orally.

Q: Which diseases can be remedied by orin therapy?

A: Orin is your body's perfect medicine and not a manmade medicine (as taught by the medical industry) for any disease. It is a means provided by one's nature to keep up the health of the body and cure the host or body, you, of any dis-ease regardless of personal beliefs.

As such, there are no limits conditions that orin cannot heal. It is only the mind that creates difficulties or impossible tasks for our ability to heal the body.

Orin is a natural auto-vaccine that's acts as an immune modulator that is very specific and personal. Auto-vaccine is defined by *The Medical Dictionary* as: "A vaccine prepared from cultures of organisms or a virus from the patient's tissues or secretions."

The antigen urinary in the orin of the patient, a natural protein that the body eliminates, has no risk or side effects and can be taken in combination with other natural resources, allowing us to slowly reduce and eliminate the inmunosupressors and chemotherapy medications that are being prescribed.

We have the ability to create our own vaccine. All the microorganisms that infect our systems from toxins and endotoxins, stimulates our immunologic system to form antitoxins (antidotes), which are discarded in the orin.

When we take it, we force the bacteria to take their own toxins, that is why we say "poison kills poison."

Orin Therapy acts as an auto-vaccine that has the same elements of our own illness (homeopathic model). It has an antiviral action, antineoplastic, antispasmodic, diuretic, anti-allergenic, anticonvulsive, and cardiovascular stimulant, anti inflammatory, anticeptic, bactericide and antifungal as well.

Q: Do you mean that even a diagnosis is unnecessary?

A: Correct. Diagnosing any disease is unnecessary. UT itself traces out the disease in the manner the police search out a thief in hiding and turns them in.

Q: Can you give an example or two?

A: Let's clarify the point by illustrating a historic fact. Perfect health is essential in yoga practices; otherwise, concentration is likely to be disturbed by bodily disorders. Even mild attacks are likely to disturb meditation. It is therefore essential that a practitioner of yoga be free from all physical troubles.

How to accomplish it?

The mystics of India, using intuition or wisdom from long experience, found out that the sure cure of orin were remarkable for all health complaints or concerns.

Q: It is wonderful, but why was this philosophy that was so beneficial and trusted, been kept a secret until now?

A: This old philosophy and cure never disappeared at all. It has been all around us and is still here; but our modern prejudiced mentality did not allow AUT to be understood or discussed, up until now. Insects, birds, fish and quadrupeds are already using this means instinctively.

By now, you've seen YouTube videos of orangutans, reindeer, camels, or giraffes drinking their pee straight into their mouths.

Only human beings, intoxicated by their intellectual power, have neglected it. They are using their skills and knowledge mainly for selfish ends.

Chapter 5
Research and clinical studies

All human beings have drank their own orin, while growing a body in the womb of their mother!

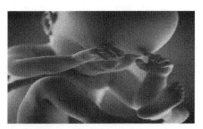

In the natural biological heaven of the human reproduction process, inside the maternal womb, is where the formation of our body took place.

The first step was the formation of mother cells, the heart, brain, kidneys, bones, basic organs, nerve cells that receives and transmit, and above all the coordination between sensorial organs and the incredible balance of genetic information, cell reproduction, and the bio-energetic stimulant.

Inside the maternal womb, we are in complete peace, comfort and harmony preparing ourselves to come out to a new life in the exterior world.

A human's perfect time on earth may be during the gestation period.

Orin Therapy is literally a gift from God (or Shiva), it is a built-in part of our nature.

There is no human on earth that has not taken his or her own orin. In our first 24-30 days, we will start peeing into the amniotic liquid!

Through the umbilical cord, the baby does receive special nutrients such as immunoglobulin and vitamins, but most of all oxygen from the mother.

When the baby reaches the age of 5 months, they urinate from 400-500 ml. Each day inside the amniotic sac, and between 8 to 9 months the baby urinates 20 to 30 times every 24 hours.

98% of the composition of the orin is water. 1% is elements consisting of cells and filaments, and the other 1% is made up of more than 1000's of healing chemical substances in the form of ions (electrically charged atoms).

Powerful substances found in milligrams, that carry the genetic information and energy of what works well or not in the body.

A fetus swallowing its own orin is not only sterile and safe; it is essential for proper biological development. A decrease in fetal orin production or excretion can result in a reduced amount of amniotic fluid.

The orin that a baby produces in utero doesn't pose any risks, even when the fetus consumes its piss. It's not only normal, but also healthy for a baby's body to run organ system functions, as well as develop swallowing, breathing and other actions needed for thriving.

Your body creates an ideal environment that protects the baby as it develops. Temperature control, nutrients, stem cells, antibody protection, and more are just a few of the automatic benefits a baby gets in the womb.

The germ situation isn't comparable to, for example, a toddler putting anything they find in their mouths.

While floating inside the womb in their orin and amniotic fluid, babies open their eyes and can see light from the outside.

Although a baby's eyes can "see" light starting around week 16, their peepers aren't fully formed until about week 20. The eyes first open between week 26 and 28.

Their vision is rather blurry, but they can see — and respond with a flutter of activity to — bright sources of light like the sun or a flashlight pointed at a woman's belly.

Thanks to pee getting into their ears, as their hearing develops, babies can hear more than we realize.

Babies are bathing their eyes in orin and observing their water world with open eyes.

While using this time to learn how to breathe and use their lungs, babies snort amniotic fluid filled with orin up their nose. It's thought they can smell food, too.

We already have experience-drinking orin through the nose from the beginning of our lives and just forgot.

Mom, getting outside helps a baby's eyes develop and reduce the risk of a few eye disorders.

When you drink or topically apply orin, you take in your own free auto-vaccine. Unlike any manmade vaccine, orin has no side effects, harmful chemicals or toxic materials in it.

In other words, orin is part of the beginning of life and we literally grew up with it built into our nature. It is a wonderful cycle of life that should never be interrupted.

Nobody can live without water.

For that reason water is a sacred element.

Nobody can live without air.

For that reason air is a sacred element.

Nobody can live without fire.

For that reason fire (including the sun) is a sacred element.

Nobody can live without taking the orin inside the mother.

For that reason orin is a sacred element.

The medical applications of orin and its constituents have been tested, discussed, researched and utilized to such an extent throughout the twentieth century that it seems incredible that almost none of us, including the majority of our doctors and medical administrators have ever heard anything about it.

But again, the reason for this is not entirely a mystery. Even though the success of urine therapy was reported long before the 1900's, 20th century medical researchers, doctors and the public turned their interests away from traditional natural medicines.

Shivambhu & Yoga are Rejuvenating

"AUT is the perfect medical solution for the millions of Indians who cannot afford medical treatment. I have been practicing it on multiple occasions, it is a profound medicine. Actually it is one of the ancient yogic techniques called Amroli Kriya. Shivambhu and yoga if practiced together, is very effective and rejuvenating." —George Fernandes, Former Defense Minister, Government of India

Orin Therapy was moved out of the home and doctor's offices and into the oblivion of research laboratories; where, unfortunately, it is being stored until the world is ready to hear about it.

UT largely disappeared from public use at the turn of the 20th century. The knowledge of the therapy is currently hidden in medical journals and research reports that people and doctors in general never see. Orin ingredients are simply isolated and converted into unrecognizable medicines and cosmetics.

Even though there have been amazing scientific discoveries about the therapeutic use of orin, medical researchers, for the most part, do not tell the public about their discoveries.

Again, this situation is most likely the result of two factors.

1. Modern medical researchers are primarily oriented towards finding strong, monetarily profitable chemical "magic bullets" to cure "symptoms" (not the cause) of specific diseases – and not towards discovering natural medicines, which augment the body's natural capacity to heal.

2. Most medical researcher's must answer to Big Pharma and are contractually bound not to reveal the results of their research until the research can become a profit-making medical therapy; patented by the company who funded the research.

Also, medical researchers tend to devote their research to extremely specialized branches of medicine, and these separate departments of medicine don't generally communicate their findings to departments outside of their own research fields.

So the urologists, for instance, who discovered that orin prevents and heals urinary tract infections might publish their findings for other urologists, but a doctor in general practice would probably not come in contact with these studies on the importance of orin in bladder or kidney infections.

The public and most practicing doctors today consider orin to be nothing more than a body waste. But *many medical researchers know that in reality, orin is an enormously comprehensive and powerful medical substance.*

Now you get to read what many scientists and doctors know, but haven't told us about the amazing curative effects of orin therapy with its anecdotal stories of healing and survival.

Regardless if orin is being generally ignored, ridiculed or written off as another "theory," people are learning the Truth and reading healing stories that are taking on significance that not even doctors can ignore.

Chapter 6
The whole body/mind connection way to supercharge AUT effectiveness through optimum diet, attitude, emotions, and self-love practices

Why does UT works for some and not for everyone?

Healing is more complex than just purifying or detoxing the physical body. Improving the diet, fasting, cleansing, right thinking or mental attitude, healthy emotions, and spiritual practices increase Shivambhu's benefits and results.

Health is result of the balance of all 4

pillars that hold together the foundation of health that a client must achieve to produce permanent well-being.

Understand? People who are miserable or self-destructive have much more work to do on themselves than do grateful, joyous folks.

Self-motived people do really well with Orin Therapy.

A well-trained or intuitively sensitive UT teacher will make inquiries into every area of a client's life in order to design a well rounded program to accelerate, deepen and secure results. *Detailed questioning is more thorough than just advising clients to do UT protocols and wishing them well.*

By taking the time to do follow-ups will bring added confidence and reassurance to the client as you work together as a team to change, improve and save a life.

Shivambhu is the gift of health

The human body requires a balance of all 4 pillars of health and wellness in order to achieve and maintain its health and longevity. The mental, emotional, physical, and spiritual aspects have to be working as one team for vitality and energy to work at its optimum. Illness can occur when a person is only focusing on some but not all of these aspects of health and well-being.

When making inquiries with clients, the compiled information will let you not only determine which direction to guide the session, but also how to make general treatment suggestions and a program that includes all of these health aspects of health.

What and how well we eat affects the color, smell, texture, and taste of Orin. Those people consuming a raw vegan or fruitarian diet tend to have clearer, tastier, and more aromatic-smelling orin than do meat, dairy, or processed food eaters. This also includes those using alcohol and prescribed or recreational drugs.

Orin is also affected by your state or mind or emotions throughout the day, especially during meals, snacks, or drinking fluids.

Reminder: You get sick either from what you eat or what's eating you?

Normal pH is within the range of 6 to 7 with an average of 6.2. A diet high in protein from meat and dairy, as well as cooked, processed or altered foods, alcohol, caffeine and drugs will not only lower the pH into a more acidic state, it will also increase the amount of mucus in the body, blood and orin (*Source: Wikipedia).

Anyone who is serious and committed to achieving their best health will do everything possible to reclaim their biological terrain (intestines and mind). The daily practice of Orin Therapy is only as effective (in your self-healing) as you are in cleaning up your diet, mind, and internal world.

Simply drinking and applying Orin *will bring results*, yet at a much slower pace when the body has to constantly do house cleaning from poor food and lifestyle choices, which is causing obstructions to vitality, strength, and energy.

Orin Therapy becomes 100 times more therapeutic as you move closer to a living plant foods and/or a fruit-based diet.

Anyone going through transitional diet changes on the way to thriving on living plant foods, adding these will boost overall healing. Consider including looping or drinking more orin daily, frequent orin enemas, fasting on orin, orin massages, and saturation dosing along with *much-needed rest*. Then you will achieve your health goals much faster.

Chapter 7
UT protocols. Introducing saturation dosing, sip looping, and new protocols discovered between 2019-2020

WARNING:

It is generally not recommended to combine orin therapy with the use of (prescribed) chemical, allopathic medicines or recreational drugs. The combination may be dangerous to your health. Why take the risk? Wait 1-2 hours before or 30-60 minutes after eating or taking medications to consume orin. Begin with the topical or external applications of AUT until you are free of all medication, if possible.

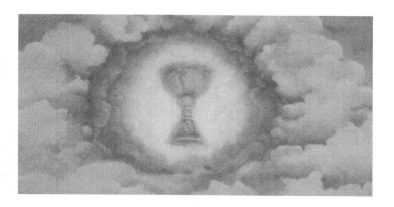

Orin Therapy Protocols

Shivambhu is a free all-purpose self-care medicine.

Make orin your default answer to any and all health concerns or conditions. Remind yourself that you carry Shivambhu in a secret container (bladder) in a body that speaks a language that just the two of you can understand.

Returning the healing water from your source back to your source will insure a long, healthy, and joyous life, indeed.

Build a lifestyle that will keep you young and healthy for your entire life by practicing UT protocols every day.

"The Shivambhu lifestyle is a labor of love"

Ask any healthy, vibrant, and devoted Shivambhu enthusiast why they are happy and well. They will exclaim with great passion in their voice, "I am blessed with health and aliveness because I drink my water."

A glass of pee a day keeps the doctor away. L'Chaim!

1. Oral Application of Orin, not only addresses all diseases, orin makes a perfect rejuvenating tonic.

As a baby step, place some drops or dropper full of orin under the tongue. Or ask client to dip a finger in some of their collected orin and then lick the orin off their finger.

This will help them form a positive association with drinking orin. They now have a wonderful natural antibiotic and remedy for anything!

The more you drink of your water, the better you feel

Beginners who start by taking little sips of Orin through the day will soon be comfortable drinking more of their water. They are often amazed how quickly they feel their energy and clarity of mind return.

The **DEFINING MOMENT** happens when one realizes that *Shivambhu is the real thing*! They have seen the light and are motivated by the possibility of achieving their health goals and a wonderful life.

Simply increase the quantity of each orin drink as you make your way to a 6-ounce (or larger) size drink of refreshing water.

It is one of the best remedies for killing pathogens, virus, fungus, and parasites in the gut and body, which in turn frees us from food slavery and all addictions.

Drinking protocols

Taking orin orally does not worsen or increase any health conditions. There is a slim chance it might be very mild and unrecognizable. When we drink fresh orin in any considerable quantity, especially in the initial months of starting UT, it may create diarrhea like symptoms, which soon heals.

Simply stop for a day. Switch to topical

protocols for this day off.

Then start drinking orin again in smaller doses, like 3-5 ounces. Increase the proportions when you feel that its ok to do so.

Oral application of Orin is a generally accepted practice. For anyone serious about reclaiming and regenerating their health quicker, *saturation dosing* (explained in next protocol) will make all the difference between feeling okay sooner than later and feeling like your healthy self again.

Newbies (anyone new to drinking pee) appreciate baby steps when starting Orin Therapy because of the mental adjustments they are making in order to accept the possibility that doing this may be good for them.

How to teach and coach newbies will be discussed in detail later in this chapter.

In addition to drinking Orin, everyone who builds a habit of practicing their favorite protocols every day can experience and discover how in combination they can receive maximum benefits and a quicker recovery.

You can either practice the same protocols every day or try different protocols every other day until you get really comfortable and experienced with them.

Perhaps you will be the discoverer of a new protocol.

By practicing and mastering the protocols it becomes easier to introduce and explain them to others.

With a lifetime of confusing, misinforming and ridiculous food rules with its dogma, no wonder why so many are obsessed, neurotic, addicted and anxious about what and how to eat right for their body.

Taking a break from eating (known as fasting) based on family/society/religious/medical/media programming around food, eating by the clock, or not learning how to know true hunger from emotional or psychological hunger gives you a mental vacation from concerns and anxiety about food.

Freeing the mind from worry about nutritional needs, medicine, healing, and creating the energy and strength for health and aliveness liberates you from obsessiveness around food, medicine, and all external forms of nourishment.

This is where you come in and sensitively teach them a new food path along with UT practices and purification techniques to empower them to enjoy life again.

"Ready to experience your best health ever by drinking pee and practicing various disciplines to treat the body/mind/spirit?"

Now it's time to grab your free personal, custom-made medicine and get the most benefits possible from Orin Therapy.

The joy and return to good health by drinking your pee starts right here and right now

Go take a whiz, then collect your water in a glass, jar, cup or bowl. Take a breath. Give thanks for what you are about to drink and for Orin delivering every vital nutrient when it is best needed for restoring your health. Enjoy.

Before going into the details with a client and teaching the protocols, here are some basics to learn before giving consultations and guiding sessions or suggesting applications for any illness.

Beginners drink 1 to 4 ounces of fresh orin in the morning or split up throughout the day. The orin can be pure or mixed with juice or distilled water.

Advanced practitioners drink 4 to 6 ounces of orin every morning (or anytime of the day) for 1 to 2 months. Work up to drinking this amount three times a day.

Work up to drinking at least 6 ounces of orin 3 times a day. Drink the beginning orin on an empty stomach first thing in the morning. Orin drinking during the day should be done at least 45 minutes before meals or up to an one hour after eating.

Spreading the time between food or medication and consuming orin will prevent indigestion or negative reaction when orin catches up with undigested food.

Practice drinking plenty of orin during intermittent fasting periods (not eating from sundown to noon) and then increase this length of time until you are fasting only on orin and distilled water (optional when looping the orin) for 24 hours at a time.

Continue the orin fast for 2 to 3 days or until you feel well.

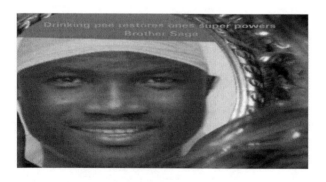

**Dr. Bunmi Sunmoila,
UT Therapist of Nigeria**

Evolve (some call "aged or maturing orin," will be explained in detail later in this chapter) orin for 4 days and try drinking 3 or more ounces on an empty stomach anytime of the day.

Using 4 days as a measurement to determine orin to be "aged" came from a theory by John W. Armstrong, author of *The Water of Life*.

Drink 2 to 4 ounces of fresh Orin every time you get a craving for the substance(s) you abuse, especially food.

Find how simply drinking orin when you get hungry can curve the appetite and take the hunger sensation away.

Fertility

Trying to get pregnant? The best and safest method is to start orin therapy for 6 months before trying to conceive and use it moderately during the days that you're attempting to conceive. You can use orin diagnostic tests to determine when you're ovulating and when you've conceived, and you can gear your use of orin accordingly.

The use of urine therapy during pregnancy

Although pregnant women are being treated successfully using UT for morning sickness or edema, some teachers believe that UT should not be used during the pregnancy without the supervision of a doctor familiar with the medical use of urine.

Concerned about the natural release of toxins that may occur with orin therapy at this time? You can choose to honor your concerns and feelings and avoid UT during pregnancy. *Or trust the innate intelligence of the body and Shivambhu and sail right through it.*

Children

There have been several research studies that deal specifically with the treatment of children using Orin Therapy. Oral drops or spoonfuls of the child's own fresh orin are considered as the easiest internal form of the therapy for children.

For acute flu, colds, viral infections, measles, mumps, chicken pox, etc., small frequent oral doses (every 2 hours) of 4 to 10 drops or 1 to 2 tablespoons during an illness have shown to be very effective. For allergies, the research studies indicate that several drops of fresh orin should be given orally before and after meals containing allergenic foods, or when allergic symptoms are present.

If the child agrees to eat only raw foods, especially fruit, during a healing or cleansing period, the results will be quicker. This eating lifestyle will keep children from experiencing the unpleasant symptoms of a headache, nausea, gas from acidosis or poor food combining, constipation, and inflammation.

Ultimately, raising children on living foods and AUT has proven to produce disease free children who grow up healthier than children who eat like everyone else.

Navel soaks are excellent for treating allergic reactions.

Another very effective method is to prepare a homeopathic dilution of the child's orin to use throughout the illness or allergy attack. Collect orin at the onset of symptoms and begin UT protocols immediately. As the body begins internal cleansing at its deepest level (or greatest threat to its well-being), symptoms of an illness may temporarily increase immediately following the first few doses of UT, but, in all cases, these symptoms dissipate within 24 to 48 hours.

For ear infections, fresh, warm orin drops in the affected ear can give excellent and often instantaneous results. Repeat as needed.

Pets and Urine Therapy

Veterinarians have given research tests on animals using urine medically by administering orin orally and topically with reportedly good results.

Night Sipping

The practice of taking a sip of orin when you wake up during the night (to pee). This is easy when you get into the habit of leaving your orin container by the bedside.

It's a time-saver, especially when you are not quite awake to coordinate body movements and have to find the way to the bathroom, just keep your orin jar on the nightstand by the bed.

Next time you get up in the night to pee, save the output, take a sip and go back to sleep. Doing this adds extra nutrients, especially melatonin, serotonin and DHEA into your body during its nighttime rest and regenerating cycle.

Swishing or Gargling

This protocol prevents bacterial over-growth by cleaning away any toxic buildup in the mouth, tongue and gums.

Pour orin in the mouth and swish it around teeth, gums and tongue. Hold a mouth full of orin for a couple of minutes. Swallow. Gargle with orin several times a day or every time you pee or think about it.

Gargling orin is good for a toothache, tongue, gums, throat ache and all ailments of the mouth.

Pulling

This is similar to coconut oil pulling. After gargling and swishing orin around the mouth, hold it in the mouth for as at least for 5 minutes. Swallow.

Looping

Looping is the practice of repeatedly drinking orin for the entire day. By looping orin, you gain the benefits from the recycling and refiltering of the dense micronutrients, reproduction of trillions of new stem cells and antibodies.

When eating while looping, it's less stress on the body to eat foods moderately that consist of living foods and/or fruit.

The advantage of looping (during an orin fast) over other forms of fasting, including water fasting, is that you get more and denser nutrients than juice or water fasting. Orin is the most nutritionally dense, bioavailable, absorbable and activated living water in the world.

You do not come out of a fasted state, which gives you the advantages of the water only fast.

Your body does not have to stop cleansing and healing. Your body increases human growth hormone (HGH) by 2,000% along with many other beneficial substances with similar increases that occur during fasting.

Every human being has already been drinking and looping pee for most of the 9 months they are in the womb—growing in a water world filled with piss and amniotic fluid. As a baby you naturally pee into the space you are floating in and drink or snort it down again; round and round it goes.

If, according to the medical system, orin is waste material, as we have been lead to believe was true, then after spending 9 months drinking our pee, snorting orin, floating in orin and growing a baby body in amniotic fluid, *every* baby would be born sick or dead.

Sip Looping

Taking a sip of fresh orin or as much as you can comfortably hold in your mouth, *every time you collect your water is called sip looping.*

Some consider this sip of pee as a dose or serving size of their medicine. This is a great way to make and keep the commitment to achieving radiant health by supplying the body with what it needs to heal you on a regular, "timed" basis.

Instead of wondering if you met the body's nutritional requirements by drinking orin, Sip looping will cover you. Does "Sip Looping" (a term coined by Doc Mike Witort*, a veteran UT Therapist of Chicago) remind you of time released pills that folks would take to get well?

This is the brilliance of sip looping. Pee. Sip. Wait for it. Pee. Sip. Repeat.

It's a no brainer. Even a newbie can do sip

looping and, after learning this UT protocol once, they are set for life.

As your body gathers all the energy and information it needs (from what you ate, what's eating you, any compromising in your systems or functions, your emotions, and how you are managing your energy), it masterfully blends the perfect elixir of immortality for you to drink and in the most perfect timing.

Combining sip looping during fasting (a water or juice fast) or when eating raw foods or fruit creates a better environment for the functions of the body's absorption, assimilation, and elimination systems.

Be sure to save the entire orin output from the day. This supply adds up quickly when practicing sip looping. You will be using this collected supply for all UT protocols.

Begin storing and evolving half of this precious water supply to use in the coming days, weeks, months or years ahead.

The other half of this supply will be used in the practices of your favorite topical protocols.

2. Saturation Dosing with AUT

The practice of increasing the oral and/or topical uses of orin.

"The saturation point" is an arbitrary attempt to reach orin capacity at its fullest or limit. Saturation dosing is your best prevention and defense of an illness or a compromised immune system. It gives you a fighting change to get ahead of any virus, sickness, contamination, or compromise to your health.

Saturation dosing is gaining in popularity as a preventative protocol, especially when started before the onset of any illness.

Considering that the body is continually regenerating and purifying itself, it's an oxymoron to believe that we could ever reach the point of being full to the max with nutrients from orin.

Keep in mind that orin, with its 3,000+ identified micronutrient-sized substances—and more yet to be discovered—it would be virtually impossible to determine "daily minimum requirements" and a "serving size" for everyone.

This is why it is clearly understood that Orin Therapy is an intuitive medicine or water.

The purpose of saturation dosing is to flood the bloodstream, body, and cells with the maximum concentration of vital nutrients in a shorter time than it takes with just one glass or serving per day.

It has been a widely held belief and practice that a glass a day of orin meets the average person's minimum health needs.

Why stop there?

This may be the case for those UT devotees who have been drinking and applying orin for many years with the addition of other health practices, like fasting, fruitarianism, raw veganism, enemas or colonics, QiGong, Tai Chi, meditation, sungazing, OMAD (one meal a day), exercise, daily conscious deep connected breathing, clearing limiting beliefs, and getting lots of hugs and conversations that matter.

Committed health enthusiasts who are continually using the UT protocols, have gained an experience and a knowing with AUT that gives them great certainty in its healing power.

Those just starting AUT using minimum doses, are improving at a snail's pace, "playing it safe," often not changing anything about their diet or lifestyle and experiencing incremental health improvement.

Education and experience using AUT is a major influence and source of inspiration for the practice and results.

AUT teachers or authors may not have taught them anything different. So, now would be a great time to bring saturation dosing into the conversation with your water buddies.

It's a great time for you and all students of this manual (and of AUT) to start practicing saturation dosing and/or increasing what you are doing with Orin Therapy until you have a direct experience of this protocol. Having the understanding and confidence in teaching this UT model to others will make a big difference for them.

This choice brings days of feeling good and days of not feeling well with varying degrees of feelings in between.

To experience a quantum leap in healing and reclaiming your well-being requires discipline, motivation, courage and faith in your self as well as the process.

How to begin UT saturation dosing

Start by putting aside all of your concerns about increasing the consumption of orin.

Trust the teachings in this manual and give 100% of your determination and energy into succeeding with AUT.

Scheduling dates and times and designing a plan of action helps when you see it laid out on a calendar for daily and weekly use. Or print out something like this one below and write in the protocol details.

SUNDAY	MONDAY	TUESDAY	WEDNESDAY	THURSDAY	FRIDAY	SATURDAY

Schedule date, time, protocol or task and duration of each protocol for each day of the week and month. Seeing this makes it real and inspires you to stay focused on the work and the goal of healing. Calendars can be motivators.

Storage suggestions for Orin

1. Choose the best container to store the water. The Damar Tantra tradition recommends the use of pots

made of gold, silver, copper, brass, iron, glass, earth or clay, bamboo, bones, leather or a bowl made of plantain leaves.

2. What to use as a cover. Cheesecloth, nylon stocking or flax/hemp sprouting type nut milk bag or even screwing on lid all works fine. Whichever cover you choose to store the orin will still result in a high quality evolving Orin.

3. Hint: Since Orin has antibacterial, antiseptic, antifungal and antiviral properties, choosing to cover or not to cover an Orin jar is a personal choice. Covering orin keeps airborne pathogens, bugs or insects from contaminating the water.

4. Drinking orin anytime of day is the best time to have a drink. Shivambhu is an intuitive medicine. It is designed into perfection for each of us. Drink as much as you can whenever you can.

5. Be sure to clean up the diet, getting closer to eating living plant foods and fruit is best. The sooner you make the change, the better.

3. Foot and Hand soaks

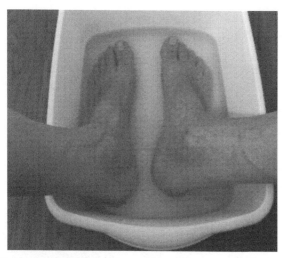

Foot and hand soaks support the over-all health of the body. These are useful for any irritation, fungus or infections of the feet, diseases, cuts, stings, bites, or eczema. Foot soaks are good for nourishing all bodi-ly functions from endocrine, digestion, ab-sorption, nervous system, lymph glands and elimination.

Place enough orin (2-4 quarts will do) in a two-gallon "Tupperware" type soft plastic square tub to cover both feet up to the an-kles.

Get barefoot. Wear loose-fitting pants, shorts, rolled-up yoga pants, pajama bot-toms, or a swimsuit. Clothing is option-al when doing a foot soak while sitting on the edge of the bathtub or on a seat in the tub. You'll be soaking for 30 minutes. Take advantage of this time by doing something relaxing or healing for you. Turn on music, sing, meditate, chant, draw, or read a book.

Use this soaking time to apply reflexology to the points on the bottom of the feet and/or hands to activate and open energy pathways for healing in every point.

It doesn't matter whether you studied reflexology or not.

Love and intention makes the orin magic work.

The pores in the bottoms of the feet have the widest openings (pores) in the entire surface of the skin. This offers maximum absorption of the orin into the blood stream. (**Orin Foot Soak Demonstration:** http://www.facebook.com/brothersage/videos/10155387211476529)

Reflexology, a healing modality that is often combined with the application of essential oils, teaches the use of touch with a certain pressure on the feet and hands to stimulate and clear the flow of energy connected to each point.

By applying orin to the soles of the palms of the hands or feet, which have the widest opening of pores on the body, the perfect medicine is instantly absorbed through the skin and transported through the blood stream and cells.

Remember to suggest the foot soak method to those hesitating to take their first sip or drink of pee.

While the feet are soaking in the golden plasma water, use this opportunity to rub or dab orin on the calves, shins and knees or as far up the legs as possible.

This same protocol is used for doing hand soaks except with a smaller sized container.

Have fun during foot or hand soaking time. You're worth it!

Excellent for treating fungus, infections, arthritis, all skin problems on the feet and hands, as well as other health conditions throughout the whole body.

4. Enemas, douches and implants

Any well-trained nutritionist, naturopath or wellness practitioner knows that to restore your body to wholeness and balance, getting started on a series or colonics or enemas should be done ASAP!!

For a chronic illness or for an occasional intestinal or body cleansing, orin enemas are a lifesaver. Administering an orin enema is a good way to remove poisonous substances from the body.

Taking orin douches for vaginal discomfort, pain or health conditions works wonders as the orin saturates the area, gets absorbed into the blood stream and brings relief. The nutrients contain anti-bacterial, anti-candida, anti-fungal & anti-cancer properties.

Orin enemas are a good way to prevent the destruction of hormones by gastric juices, build up of toxic material and obstruction or congestion, which is why this method often helps to cure allergic disorders better. This is also true for orin injections.

Furthermore, a number of compounds in orin are better absorbed this way then by oral ingestion.

Many people will prepare a filled plastic or glass gallon container with full strength or dilluted orin before starting a series of enemas. This will give you enough orin to give yourself 3 to 4 rounds of enemas.

Remove rugs from bathroom. Lay a beach towel size towel on the bathroom floor. Hang filled enema bag on a drawer handle, towel rack or toilet paper fixture. Be sure you have locked the clamp on the lower end of the tube before you hang up the bag to prevent spills.

Test the temperature of the orin before pouring it into the enema bag to determine if adding hot water would be more comfortable without the initial mild shock of inserting tube with cold orin up the bum. Adding extra hot water (tap water is fine) to the enema bag helps the gut and body to relax. You will feel more comfortable during the process.

A single massage oil, like sesame (avoid oil blends that contain volitile oils like cinnamon or peppermint that will sting in a very sensitive area), is poured on the tip of the enema tube to lubricate it for easier insertion. When finished with enema, be sure to allow time for deep cleaning of all surfaces of the toilet, floor and bathroom sink area as well as the enemas bag and attachments.

Put aside time after an enema to relax, rest and recharge your energy.

Next step after filling the lower intestine with orin. While sitting on the toilet, hold in the orin in the colon for as long as possible before letting it go.

Optional: After the material is discharged, apply fresh or evolving orin on the skin of the entire body.

Optional: Get into a tub filled with hot water,

as hot as you can stand it. Stay in it for up to 20 minutes. After that go to the bed and cover with a few blankets if needed to sweat out a fever.

Taking orin douches for vaginal discomfort, pain or health conditions works wonders as th,e Orin saturates the area while purifying the vagina of pathogens and toxins as it is getting absorbed into the blood stream to bring relief.

Douche with fresh or evolving orin.

The nutrients as well as the antibacterial, anticandida, antifungal, and anticancer properties in Orin are the quickest, safest and most effective way to eliminate pathogens, parasites, yeast, candida, fungus, tumors, discharge and unhealthy bacteria.

Try inserting 3 to 6 ounces of orin in the colon and hold it in as long as possible. This is called a rectal implant. These 3- to 6-ounce silicon or soft rubber bulbs are sold at pharmacies, health food stores, or online.

It can be taken anytime. This is a quick way to introduce orin into the colon without the lengthy process of set up, use and clean up from an enema.

A cleanse is even better when a rectal implant is done after bowel movement.

5. Ears

Rinse the ears with orin from either the palm of your hand or use a dropper to apply orin drops in the ears. While head is tilted to the direction opposite the side of the filled ear, massage or pull along the inner edges of the ear to encourage the orin to sink deeper into the ear.

Got ear health challenges? Squeeze a dropper full of orin into inner ear canal (Eustachian tube) with your head lying down on the opposite side.

Hold orin in ears for as long as you can. Try leaving it in an ear for 5 minutes. When ready, tilt head to opposite side and let it drain. Repeat protocol with the other ear.

Use orin ear rinses to treat hearing, tinnitus or any ear infections.

An alternative method to eardrops is to place an orin soaked cotton ball in the ear(s). Keep in the ear for one hour, and then remove it. Tip head to the side of the ear and massage throughout the ear to either absorb or drain the remaining orin.

Q-tips are useful, not only in applying and dabbbing orin inside the ears, but they can also be used in other ways. Most people will easily sniff a finger dipped in pee as a beginner's method of drinking orin through the nose. While others prefer the use of a Q-tip to swab orin on the inside of both nostrils to clean out bacteria and the nasal passage, as they lightly sniff the orin.

This is a personal choice.

Q-tips, like cottonballs soaked in orin, work well for a quick remedy for specific conditions. However, in any emergecy situation, like a hornet or wasp sting, burn or cut, you'll need to move quickly on an AUT treatment.

Forget about rushing home or scrambling though the medicine cabinet or bathroom drawers for supplies. Either pee directly on any affected areas or pee in the palm of a hand to transfer to anywhere on the body.

6. Eye rinse

Obtain a eye cup from local drug store, healthfood store or online. Fill up eye cup with fresh orin to avoid a sting from the astringent quality of evolving orin. Press and hold firmly to one eye. Blink several times while cup of orin is still secure.

Pour excess orin remaining in the cup directly over the eye and surrounding area.

—Dr. Roslynn Hansen

Then switch eye cup and repeat protocol with the other eye.

The eye rinse protocol supports eye health, bringing relief to tired, burning or painful eyes. Use orin ear rinses to treat all irritation, cataracts, poor vision, swimmer's eyes, sore or tired eyes or any eye infections.

"To treat any type of eye problems, do the following:

Drink fresh orin into both nostrils from time of awakening until 6 p.m. After 6 p.m., collect all orin until bedtime. This orin shall be collected for external uses (i.e., pour into eyes 3 to 4 times a day). Give youself an orin body massage from someone or from yourself in the next few days. It shall prevent and treat many other diseases such as coronavirus." —Dr. Rakshak Mal Lodha

Make certain that the eyedropper you use for eye rinses is sterilized. A compress of fresh orin is also excellent for external eye inflammations such as styles.

7. Orin Fasting: the ultimate choice in purification

Question: How does one go on an Orin fast?

Answer: Fasting is a conscious vacation from food. It is a yoga of mindfulness with attention on the body and mind during a cleansing and rebuilding time and not on eating.

Collect and drink up to 100% of your orin shortly after peeing. Drink only orin (or combine with distilled water) for the entire day. Drink enough orin to satiate your thirst. To overcome hunger sensations throughout the day, drink 2 to 3 ounces.

Notice that the hunger left.

The advanced fasting practice is to drink as little orin as possible for the day. This puts you on the edge of a dry fast.

It is extremely powerful and effective.

Avoid drinking orin or any fluids a couple of hours before bedtime; otherwise, your sleep may be disrupted by trips to go pee.

Two hours before bedtime, take a break from drinking orin, collect and save your orin in a large sized glass container, like a 2-quart glass "Ball or Mason" jar.

Use this orin for all cosmetic (some call topical) uses or oral applications for the next day or over the next few weeks (or longer to allow it to continue evolving).

Patience (yes this means you, too) is required when drinking all the orin that you are peeing during the day.

Since you drink your pee and have read this far into this Manual, *you earned a Peequent flyer award.* Notice if you feel like your peequency is at a higher vibration.

Orin becomes clearer, neutral in its smell and sweeter on the day you fast.

1. Orin fasts have no limits on what health conditions it can improve. Orin fasting works quicker when combined with other natural, adjuvant therapies.
2. Orin fasts help with dust, house dust mites,
   (1) Mold allergies, chemical allergies with or without orin injections. However, orin injections while fasting are a more rapid treatment.
3. Orin fasts increases stem cells, HGH (Human Growth Hormone), anti-bodies, probiotics, steroid hormones and their metabolites and thyroid hor-

mones.

4. Orin fasting improves intelligence, imagination, creativity, sense of humor, short-term (intermediate-term and long term) memories, and sharpens thinking abilities. Critical and "the Big Picture" thinking skills also return.

5. Orin fasting makes us feel like slowing down, taking time to meditate, feeling grateful and closer to Love.

6. As a result of Orin fasting and people making healthier lifestyle choices, more are experimenting with living foods or a fruit-based diet.

7. Orin fasting combined with the topical application of fresh or evolving orin does wonders on skin conditions as it lubricates and nourishes the skin.

8. Orin fasting is effective in treating intestinal parasites, virus, fungus, pathogens and yeasts (candida).

9. While Orin reestablishes our balance from food allergies and any form of "it-is" in the intestinal tract from exposure to pathogens from our diet and outside sources, the body will detox itself of heavy metals, drugs and chemicals (which are stored in body fat).

10. Dormant centers in the brain are acti-

vated and bring a greater appreciation of music, singing, dance, romance, art and the innumerable gifts of life.

11. Combining regular orin fasting with a living foods or fruit-based diet, exercise, meditation and rest, can make all the difference in restoring health and wellness. Conscious deep connected breathing and slowing down allows one to achieve good energy management.

12. During an Orin fast, detoxing may occur as the body is restoring its healthy bacteria in the gut.

13. Cataracts are usually removed in 10-14 days.

14. According to J.W. Armstrong, author of *The Water of Life*, a client fasted on orin for 101 days and cured his blindness.

15. Those with post-traumatic stress disorder (PTSD), Alzheimer's, senility, ADHD, ADD, Autism Specturm Disorder, or bipolar disorder and have emotional traumas report great results. This is accredited to the presence of DHEA, melatonin, serotonin, dopamine, B vitamins, oxytocin, magnesium and other important nutrients for

the glands, brain and nervous system.

16. All healing comes from within and goes out to the surface (skin), from the head down, and in reverse order as the symptoms have appeared or have been suppressed.

17. Orin becomes lighter in color and sweeter in taste with each collection and round of having drinks.

18. Orin compresses during Orin fasting applied 24/7 are wonderful for gangrene, cut, burns, insect or snakebites, sunburns and all skin conditions.

19. Take up a mucus and acid free diet (no dairy, meat, carbs or processed foods) along with Orin fasting and watch how quickly the excess mucus is eliminated. Keep extra tissues handy.

20. Enjoy better sleep and less sleep while Orin fasting.

21. Orin fasting removes heavy metals and toxins safer and faster than zeolite, wheatgrass juice, shilijit or a far infrared sauna.

22. Orin fasting repairs and cleanses all the cells of
    a. Cellular and metabolic waste, facilitating cancer,
    b. Healing and non-genetic diseases.

Practicing orin and distilled water fasts for two days a week, preferably on your days off, like Friday afternoon or Sunday afternoon, is great for healthy people. It gives the body an opportunity to heal what needs to be healed and prevent the onset of any problem.Fast for 7 days on water with lemon (adding stevia or raw honey with pinch of cayenne is optional) and orin only.

Fast for 30 days on orin and water only.

Question: How long should I do an Orin fast?

Answer: Start practicing intermittent fasting from 6 p.m. to 10 a.m. daily. Skip "breakfast." **Do a fast** of about 16 hours.

Your digestive system will thank you for the good rest. With orin, you can start with an ounce (shot glass works well for measurements). Most serious Orin drinkers will drink the entire amount that was collected. A basic Orin fast can last from 1 to 3 days.

Typically most orin fasts last 7, 14, 21, or 30 days. Some people have been known to fast beyond 30 days to heal more serious health challenges. One man fasted on the Master

Cleanse for 365 days and healed paralyzed legs. He threw away his wheelchair and takes brisk walks everyday.

Imagine what UT would have done for him.

Simply fast long enough to cure whatever dis-ease you "think" you have. Always listen, trust and follow your intuition. John W. Armstrong, the author of "The Water of Life" was known to have his patients do an Orin fast for 101 days to cure blindness in the eyes.

The mere length of orin fasting can raise human growth hormone to very high levels while fasting and correct conditions.

Soak a cotton ball or washcloth in fresh or evolving Orin. Gently dab or wipe on areas to be healed. Use for burns, sunburn, cuts, scratches, acne, bruises, capillary bursts (sudden discoloration of skin to reddish purple) and anything on general skin surfaces.

Make a compress with orin leaving area covered for hours or overnight.

You can always use a washcloth, cotton ball

or just the hands for topical applications.

Rub orin on the skin as it cleanses, rejuvenates, brings elasticity back to your cells and tones your muscles. It will leave the body in the form of sweat, pimples or skin rashes, fever or as energy.

8. An *Orin body massage, including facials, scalp, head, feet, hands and hair rubs*, are very complementary to fasting and enemas, as a treatment for skin disorders, diseased body parts, internal organs, wounds and a rejuvenating whole-body tonic. Orin makes a good substitute for soap.

Take 30 to 60 minutes to receive or give you or give to another, an orin body massage for wellbeing.

Go slowly and softly while massaging orin toward the heart. Pay attention to massage the areas where the lymph glands are located. Send kind and loving thoughts and positive energy to the recipient. Allow at least an hour for the orin to be absorbed. When orin is absorbed into the skin, the odor of ammonia will be gone after a short period of time.

Orin massages are easy to love and appreciate. It's worth it for the wonderful feeling of being healthy and invigorated.

Scalp and hair massage as a general hair care, substitute for shampoo and conditioner, dandruff or hair loss and baldness. Using fresh or evolving orin, massage orin briskly into scalp allowing it to be absorbed thirty minutes to an hour or as long as possible. Then wash it out with lukewarm water. Get ready for clean, lustrous and darker colored hair.

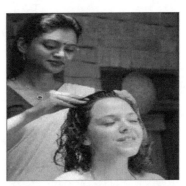

Remind your mind that you are giving and receiving a loving and nurturing massage using holy water and that you're worth it!

Best Orin Shampoo recipe

1. Find an appropriate size jar or bottle
2. Pee in the bottle
3. Apply and massage orin into your hair and scalp
4. Thrive

On a healthy diet, dried orin does not have an offensive odor.

Food Poisoning

Several research studies have show that urea is a proven antibacterial agent (Drs. Schlegel, Kaye, Weinstein etc.), and orin has been found to contain antibodies to food contaminants such as salmonella bacteria in infected individuals (Lamer and Remington). Begin by taking 3 or 5 drops. Increase dosage as tolerated from a dropper full to an ounce or more.

9. Nose drinking, sniffing or snorting

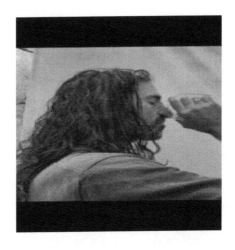

Demonstration by Samuel G Cohen*

Your best health ever may be a mere change of mind and a willingness to trust the success of many who are drinking orin through the nose and can testify to the many benefits and healings they are having.

This is how to teach others how to overcome their resistance or mind talk about this protocol. Meditate on nose drinking. Take a deep breath. Take baby steps. After dipping a finger in orin, stick it up a nostril and sniff or snort it deeply. Repeat process in other nostril.

Congratulate yourself. Then day by day

step up the quantity of orin that you sniff until you are mentally ready to drink ounces of orin through the nose.

Drinking Orin Through The Nose
© 8.2020 by Samuel G Cohen

DrinkingThroughTheNose.com

The practice of drinking through the nose protocol forms part of a unique way of life designed to awaken the brain, activate the 3rd eye and change the practitioner into a new being; "a being" who is way above what they have been known to be by the wider population.

We had read about Taoists in India using the same method with Orin therapy. Yet it was Kelly Ra Saliba who had discovered this technique while in his bathroom in London in the year 2000. Now over 20 years later, what have we come to learn? (Kelly Ra Saliba offers his teachings via DrinkingThroughThe Nose.com)

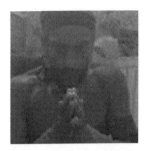

The option of ingesting fresh or mature orin opens up a whole dimension uncharted to any extensive degree. The combination of UT and Sahaja Yoga Meditation raises the Kundalini in the individual, nourishes the nervous system and awakens the chakras located within the spinal column in the Sushumna (Central Channel).

Once the Kundalini rises in a safe and secure manner, there is an opening of the 3rd eye and piercing of the Sahasrara. Only then can the adept truly drink through their nose. The nose drinking is both physiological and spiritual in equal measures.

Mantras (prayers) used during orin drinking have facilitated our practice immensely, where we have now reached the ability to drink anything through our nose, provided it is from Mother Nature.

Orin is the baby and was the first elixir we began with solely for two years up the nose. As our noses were blocked and mucus was being flushed out, we had to practice being comfortable with drinking any fluid at first.

Every person will need to practice patience when passing through this stage.

To be conscious of Taoist Lovemaking is a third way to activate the hormones, pheromones and enzymes in our vehicles. The secretions we absorb when a man and a woman join in loving union are super-healing. It feeds and nourishes our nerves and brain similar to drinking orin or specific juices, elixirs, tinctures, colloids, essences, whatever we choose up the nose as a nasal drink.

The man maintains the climax, avoiding the localized orgasm, while the woman learns to channel her orgasm. This cannot be underestimated.

So it is with Orin Therapy. Providing we are ingesting plenty of natural and nutritious raw foods, fruits, salads, veggies and hemp seeds, our orin will be a blessing for our beings on many levels.

To simply just throw out orin into a toilet (when you pee) when our vehicles are quietly aging, dehydrating, literally drying out, is a shame. As a result the body has to remanufacture itself, which could be put to use in self-healing and increasing one's wellbeing.

Once we begin drinking orin everyday through the mouth and nose including massaging orin into our skin, our circulation heightens, skin appears and feels younger and smoother. Plus our hair feels deeply nourished.

It was when we learned to respect the Tao of Lovemaking and look further into Sahaja Yoga Meditation, did we see the genuine benefits it could truly offer.

While currently being in Goa, India for 5 months, I have been blessed to learn Yoga asanas, fasting and breath work. The combination of these 3 practices has been formidable pillars that formed our already rich armory.

These have enabled me to reach further heights and plateaus with meditation, silencing the mind, increasing healing powers, deepening & strengthening love for people, animals and self-love, clearing of family relationships issues, peaceful contemplation, achieving a calming presence and an enhanced intelligence.

Allowing the Holy Spirit to be my guide has been a continual source of nourishment and a way to stay centered.

According to Samuel, *"It is impossible to get a cold when you constantly drink orin through the nose."*

"You can feel under the weather but one

drink up the nose and any clouds start to evaporate."

"I take a cup with me everywhere. If I have to go to the bathroom, I take it with me, close the door, collect my water and drink through my nose."

"*You feel like Superman*—you're going to go into a phone booth and do something nobody knows and it's a secret."

The elixir through the nose is a vital part of purifying ones waters, keeping you youthful, feeling protected, joyful and in bliss.

We hope that you can embark on this special journey of self-discovery. Bon Voyage!"
—Samuel

Nasal wash works well with the use of a "neti pot" to flush nasal sinuses or nasal cavities. The intestines in the body contain a secondary set of sinus portals and they are in charge of keeping the brain clean. Sinus problems, headaches and congestion are easily remedied with orin nasal flushes and naval soaks.

Other nasal methods that you will receive great benefit includes sniffing from the palm of hand, sniffing an orin soaked finger in each nostril, using a squirt bottle or a small 3-ounce enema type rubber bulb.

Six Forms of UT Nose Drinking

Tipping the head backwards and drinking orin down the throat while sniffing is just one form of UT nose drinking.

Here are 5 other types of nasal drinking

Before beginning, rub fresh orin in each eye, although not essential.

Begin by taking a sitting position with legs underneath almost like a squat posture placing all weight on the knees.

Tip the head down to position the top of the head on the ground in front of your knees.

Insert glass pipette or squirt bottle into first nostril and while keeping tip of head on the ground (upside down head) to ensure no orin flows out or down throat, insert 1 to 2ml of 100% pure orin.

Using Evolving orin that you have is best for this procedure.

The orin will go up your nose and travel to

behind the eye. It then enters the prefrontal cortex part of the brain which is responsible for thought processes and then makes its way to the pineal and pituitary glands.

You may wish to curse with discomfort, sneeze a lot, feel a tremendous pressure behind the eye and feel a bit of pain but this is all normal at the start.

With continued practice of nose drinking, the sinuses become rehydrated or moist and the discomfort soon passes. It is well known that *drinking or sniffing orin though the nose can decalcify and activate the pituitary gland.*

Placing your free hand on the forehead during this difficult time will support you through the process.

The other 4 forms are repeating this same method by inserting pipette and delivering 1-2ml. The difference is to have your head tilted keeping top of head on the ground, look up to the ceiling while viewing bum in the air.

This angular position will allow orin to travel into deep parts of the skull through the sinus and soft tissues. You will feel it going to the back of the ear and inside the face.

These 5 forms are with the head tipped in different positions to allow orin to reach different sites in the head and brain through the tubules and nerves inside the head.

Experiment with it to where you need it most, i.e. where the pain is most extreme.

Afterward you may feel like a head cold coming on. Allow all mucus to come up and out of the nose. Phlegm of all kinds will be discharged. You will notice that breathing air becomes significantly easier than ever before. You will feel like you have not breathed this freely since being very young.

Thinking becomes clearer and head feels lighter.

After some nose blowing, eye weeping and coughing up mucus, nose drinking becomes as natural as oral drinking.

Repeat exact procedure through the second nostril. One or two days later when you are ready, do 1st nostril procedure a second time with the 5 forms of UT nose drinking. After alot of mucus membranes have been cleared and unblocked, you will experience a cleaner and simpler type of pain (if any) with less head pressure.

Nose drinking clears up migraine headaches.

As you go deeper through the cavities of the brain, the pineal gland receives the orin much quicker. The orin will pull heavy metals from the pineal as it rehydrates this master gland.

You will not sneeze anymore after a few procedures. Even if you try it for a few days, stop for a month and try it again, you will not sneeze and the pain will be significantly reduced.

The rewards are incredible and once you see the results of the first try, you will be interested to do it again. The discomfort can be disconcerting but the good feeling is far more delightful.

Peace,

Labhaoise

10. Orin **air purification with a nebulizer, hand held respirator, humidifier or mister**

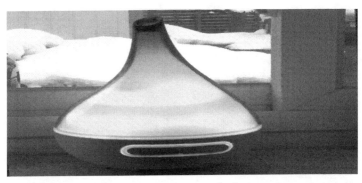

This is the easiest and least expensive method to purify a room of any airborne particulates, bacteria or virus.

Either dust off and clean your nebulizer, diffusor or humidifier or buy one. An alterative would be a clean quart size spray bottle.

Demo of Diffusing Orin with a Diffuser

Fresh orin 1-3 days old is a common age used for this protocol. Nebulizing (another way of saying misting) orin in a nebulizer results in cleaner and more alive feeling air. Try adding a few drops of lemon or orange essential oil if orin smells too pungent. Or thin down orin with distilled water.

Turn the unit on. Enjoy a room made clean and fresh by your own water. Let it run for 2-6 hours before turning it off. If you can find a nebulizer that has a light, like in this photo, enjoy the golden glow it casts. The golden glow is more profound when using full strength orin.

Respirator protocol

There are small tabletop sized respirators that work great with this protocol. Included with respirator is a tube with a mouthpiece and an optional plastic facial mask.

Simply pour orin in the chamber and cover lid. This chamber holds approximately one ounce of a fluid. Place lips firmly over mouthpiece. Turn on nebulizer motor and inhale.

To deliver your perfect medicine directly into the sinuses, master glands and brain; use the mask for inhaling nebulized orin.

Hand held air freshener

Consider this as a possibility. Find or buy a 3-5 oz. glass bottle with spray top. Fill with fresh or evolving orin. Mist face, hands, skin conditions and eyes to refresh the mind/body during long drives, walks in Nature, for a sunburn, while sitting in boring classes or lectures or any times of stress like being in the public or on any public transportation.

Keep a filled bottle in the car or backpack. Whenever the air feels stale or has unpleasant odors, use it as an air freshener/disinfectant to cleanse room or area of airborne pathogens, molds or viruses.

Carry an orin mist bottle in purse or backpack when on bus, plane, cab or train. Be sure to mist or spray the headrest and seat (on both sides if possible) you are riding in to cleanse any pathogens left by untold passengers. If riding as a passenger for a long trip, you may wish to spray your bare feet or hands in order to stay relaxed and alert.

Until one gets in the habit of collecting some of their pee while using a public bathroom to "disinfect" and wash those precious hands after peeing, using an orin mist bottle works well.

Spraying on the face, hands and feet will

nourish the body quickly as it wakes you up. Think stem cells, antibodies and regeneration of the endocrine and nervous system.

This is a great way when traveling for long periods of time to refresh both the body and mind.

Or for using anywhere you are in the public or on public transportation. Spray the orin in the bathroom, you silly readers. Did you think I meant on headrests, seats and passengers? *Does make one stop and think about actually doing this possibility.*

11. Dropper bottle filled with evolving orin

Does your energy dip during the day? Here's a proven protocol that will energize *and* calm you. Keep a closed dark amber or cobalt blue colored glass dropper bottle filled containing orin in purse or backpack. Gargle and swallow a dropper full or more anytime you need to increase your energy or regain clarity of mind. This can be a lifesaver during the day.

Plus, use this orin for emergency situations, drop and rub orin on cuts, scratches, stings, rashes, bites or sunburn.

12. **Orin Injections**

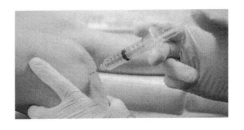

Orin injections are usually reserved for life threatening situations. These can be a life-saver when drinking orin is not possible or desired; especially useful when treating allergic reactions, shock or anxiety.

Many report positive results in a very short time. Any cleansing reaction is short-term from a day to a week.

As the body purifies, be prepared for clients who demonstrate symptoms such as these: headache, joint and muscle pain, body aches, sore throat, general malaise, sweating, chills, nausea or other symptom type of reactions that may feel very intense.

Be ready to face it and not panic or interrupt the process with any unnatural or human made medicine. Orin injections will awaken the immune system and its warriors ready for fighting any disease.

In case of emergencies, when there is no time to lose, an injection with evolving orin (the strongest effects have been noticed when using orin that has evolved several months) can save a person's life.

Your orin is always your perfect medicine.

It contains substances that your body does not need. These will aggravate the body, which causes the defense system to develop stronger antibodies for anything that would compromise or harm the body.

Injecting orin causes the body to go into a hyper active healing mode which forces it to heal and release toxins immediately.

Direct injection of orin into the blood stream will bypass the stomach, digestion and elimination systems. This makes it very potent.

New research (which is bringing needed hope) reveals that orin therapy can be beneficial under all of these conditions.

It is recommended for clients to not use orin

therapy when using any type of drugs or medication, heavily smoking (tobacco or cannabis), drinking alcohol or coffee.

An American doctor, Dr. William Hitt, who runs orin therapy clinics in Mexico, has reported treating 20,000 patients (over a 2 year period) with orin therapy injections.

These patients have included those diagnosed with cancer, asthma, heart and other diseases along with patients effected with severe alcoholism, drug and smoking addictions.

Dr. Hitt had great success with his clients with no side effects from using orin injections for addictive disorders and also in combination with prescription drugs. Lab testing showed that the amount of drugs or contaminants passed into orin was so infinitesimal that they pose no threat and, in fact, appear to act as auto-vaccine agents which improve or cure these types of disorders.

Results like this demonstrate Orin's effectiveness even when small quantities of orin are taken in moderate to diluted form like in a homeopathic or tincture form.

In the book Urinalysis in Clinical Laboratory Practice from Miles Laboratories, the authors state that even in a case of severe mercury poisoning, the actual amount of mercury passed into the orin is infinitesimal.

Teach your clients how to avoid heavy detoxification, when these types of conditions are present, by starting with *1-5 drops up to a dropperful* of orin orally per day for 3 days. Increase the dose by 5 drops each day according to how well they are tolerating the therapy; gradually increase the amount as needed to obtain results for an individual condition.

Many people have asked about the efficacy of orin injections, and as you've seen, many of the research studies presented utilized injections of orin as part of the therapy.

Ironically, doctors are also using oral orin or urea therapy in nonemergency cases with equally good results. Some patients receiving orin injections have reported a side effect of occasional redness and swelling at the site of the injection, which doesn't occur, of course, with oral therapy.

Drinking orin allows for slower application

and absorption, which can decrease any possible detoxifying symptoms. Injections deliver an abrupt, forced introduction of nutritional substances into the body, without allowing for the body's gradual adjustment to the substance.

There really isn't any need for this sudden forcing of orin into the body unless there is an emergency situation that requires it.

Orin injections work fine if you are comfortable giving these to yourself or others. Or you can consult a health expert to administer this for you.

> "My faith is strong in UT because (in addition to the books & research I have read) has improved my overall health. I was able to get off all prescription medication. My skin & eyes have benefited greatly from morning wash/rubs *and I know* it is protecting me from harmful environmental toxins as well." —Grace Purcell

13. Goggles

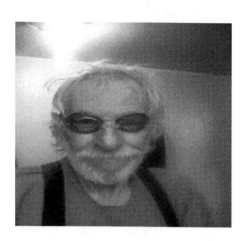

This is a simple and fun protocol for healing the eyes. Much thanks to *George Johnson for inventing this method.*

Fill up goggles with fresh orin. Using fresh orin for eye washes is more comfortable, soothing and less astringent on the eyes than using evolving orin. After filling the goggles with pee, press them against eyes, feeling for the suction to feel right, while adjusting them until you get the right fit.

Wear your water filled goggles for approximately 10-15 minutes, give or take a few minutes. Blink occasionally. Remove goggles and rub any dripping orin on the face.

Your eyes will feel fresh, new and clear

again. Rinsing eyes with water is optional.

14. Tongue cleaning

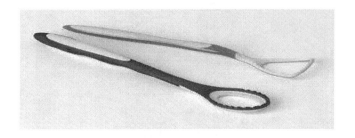

Lecture on the UT tongue
cleaning protocol* (http://www.
facebook.com/brothersage/vid-
eos/10157102159071529)

The use of a tongue cleaner that you can
get from your dentist or pharmacy. *Tongue
cleaning* is the activity of dragging a tongue
cleaner dipped in orin across the tongue.

This protocol supports oral hygiene as it
cleans off the coating that been growing (for
who knows how long) on the tongue. The
tongue collects microorganisms and oral de-
bris consisting of food, saliva and dead skin
cells. The tongue surface can store tooth and
gum pathogens. Tongue cleaning with orin

restores oral health, which directly restores blood and cellular health. This protocol removes the layer of contaminants that coats the tongue.

Repeat when coating returns or mouth feels nasty and you have bad breath. A living foods and fruitarian diet eliminates most of the oral health concerns.

Dip tongue cleaner in fresh orin.

Scrape tongue with a pulling downward motion toward tip of tongue several times until you feel complete. Or until the tongue looks pink and clean. Rinse mouth with fresh orin or water. Spitting it out is optional.

15. Navel or belly button soak

Perhaps you may have thought, why would we put orin (same idea applies to essential oils) in and on the bellybutton?

Our Navel (Nabhi) is an amazing gift that our Creator has given us. According to science, the first part that takes form after conception is the navel. After it is created, it joins the mother's placenta through the umbilical cord.

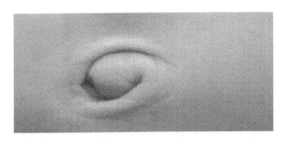

Our Navel is surely an amazing thing! All our veins are connected to our navel, which makes it the focal point of our body.

The belly button is life itself!

The "Pechoti", the bit that is left over after the umbilicus has been cut at birth, is behind the navel, which has more than 72,000 veins. The total amount of blood vessels we have in our body is equal to double the circumference of the earth.

Well, it seems that in Ayurveda, the belly button is used as a portal to deliver nutrients or medicines into the body. Now we know that all humans have a belly button unless you were born with an umbilical hernia and had to have it surgically repaired, leaving you without the navel.

But not every mammal has belly buttons. Kangaroos and platypuses are without a belly button. But dolphins are not.

Belly buttons accumulate a lot of bugs. Some 2,400 different species have been found lurking in the navel. And everyone's belly button bugs are a different composition. Navel lint is a gross mix of fibers, hair, and dead skin cells.

You may be wondering, how is the belly button so powerful? It's all about location, location, location. The belly button is near the center of your abdomen and around your center of gravity (3rd chakra, center or core).

It sits over your intestines and major lymph nodes and blood vessels. And it's near your vagus nerve, which is responsible for the rest and digestion functions of the body.

Unlike the rest of the abdomen, there's little to no muscle behind the navel, which makes it the perfect access point to your belly. The rest of the body connects to the belly button by fascial trains that cross right near it.

It's also the entry point for the major energy center in your lower abdomen. Navels are very important reflexology points that stimulate the whole body. So how can you harness the powers of your belly button?

We have known that to lower the temperature for the babies, we put a cotton swab with alcohol in the navel, now we know that with orin, it's healthier, safer and better.

Your navel can detect which veins have dried up and by putting on orin, those nerves open them.

Applying orin in the navel heals the dryness of the eyes, poor vision, the pancreas, heels, chapped lips, keeps the face bright, the hair healthier, knee pain, the chills, lethargy, pain in the joints and dry skin.

Apply Orin in your belly button

Belly Button Healing: The Secret to Health is in the Belly Button* (https://youtu.be/f88WoCxHLdl)

1. eliminates stubborn pimples and acne

2. achieve a glowing face

3. hydrates and moistens dry, chapped lips. Keeps your intestines moving while removing only harmful bacteria and keeping the good. Orin actually works as a mild detox.

4. improves fertility

5. works wonders for a cold, flu and a running nose. When a baby has stomach pain, put a few drops directly in the navel and give a gentle massage around the navel a few minutes. The pain will be gone shortly.

6. eases menstrual pain and cramps

7. reduces for all types of joint pains ("ititis"). It can strengthen bones. Parents use UT with their children every night at bedtime.

8. relieves upset stomach, bloating, nausea and digestive problems.

9. improves blood flow to the nervous system and also enhances the immunity system.

10. heals constipation and builds a strong digestive system.

11. relaxes arteries and veins, lowering blood pressure and stress to the heart. Also helps strengthen and tone the heart muscles.

12. as a diuretic, orin removes excess water, salt and toxins, overweight, blood pressure, and digestion.

13. is an expectorant that removes mucus from the airways and lungs. Orin is effective in treating bronchitis, whooping cough and upper respiratory inflammation.

At night before bed, apply 3 drops of orin in your navel and spread it 1 and a half inches around your navel. An orin soaked cotton-ball can be placed in the navel with a washcloth over it as a method to slowly drip orin into the bloodstream while sleeping.

Remember orin is a powerful compound and safe to use directly on the skin, as this does not cause sensitization and irritation. It does not have to be diluted unless a rapid detox would be of concern by a client or therapist.

Try this for tremors, strokes, lethargy, spaciness, equilibrium or dizziness concerns, depression, inflammation and dry skin.

16. Evolving Orin
The Evolutionary Urine Theory
©2020 Brother Sage

Keep in mind that orin contains information and memory of our perfect health. As the body's health becomes challenged or compromised, it does a system check or self-diagnostics to restore perfect health and balance.

Imagine what we can learn from drinking evolving orin?

Here is another paradigm shifting term to tickle your mind. The terms "evolved and evolving" have replaced the terms "aged and aging" previously used in describing, "maturing" orin (term made popular by *Monica Schütt)

Evolution, by its very nature, is a continuum of growing, learning and making discoveries. Orin, like humanity, evolves forever from the moment it arrives and is collected.

Evolution as defined by Webster's Dictionary is a process of gradual, peaceful, progressive change or development.

Do the words "aged and aging" bring comfort to your mind or make you feel uneasy in the body?

Aged and aging are words or symbols that we associate with as loss of strength, health and vitality. Discussing aging brings up images of old people who are sick, hurting, have memory loss and are dying.

This explains why people feel disgust and taken back when it is suggested that they include drinking or applying "aged" orin in their UT practices.

Try this when you are talking or writing about "aged urine." Hey, Lisa, I am so glad that you are getting results from drinking your fresh orin. You may wish to try a more potent version of orin?

Brother Sage, the Shivambhu guru, says that Evolving or Evolved Orin is an Evolutionary idea. According to his theory, every second your orin is outside of your body and sits in a container, it is increasing in potency, life force or shakti, and frequency. All collected orin comes already ACTIVATED and immediately becomes ENHANCED and AMPLIFIED, which is the evolutionary power of our water of life.

Are you drinking "common" wine or will you try the ultra refined wine of goddesses and gods!

Evolutionary Orin for the Next Generation!!

You may wish to start a client off slowly in making the change or transition to using evolving orin.

Aged vs. Fresh Orin
by Monica Schütt*
(annotated by Brother Sage)

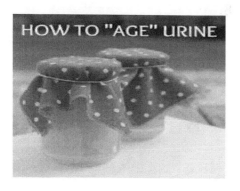

Orin is considered "aged" or made more powerful from

4 days of incubation (ref. J.W. Armstong author of the 1944 classic, The Water of Life: Treatise on Urine

Therapy).

Orin contains stem cells that multiply by the trillions

when it is left alone to incubate for days, months

or years.

Let orin sit at room temperature (any place indoors or out-doors) in an open container, covered with only a thin piece of cloth, so the orin can "breathe." This is important.

There is a special alchemical reaction happening when orin gets in contact with air/oxygen. It should be kept open for at least a couple months. Longer is better but watch out that it does not all get evaporated. FYI. Evaporated orin crystalizes into ormus powder of gold. This can keep forever. It is highly concentrated. Only a pinch is needed for a serving.

Cover with a cheese cloth, fabric or paper filter secured with rubber band, so that no dust or insects can get in. Aged orin is a very potent remedy and it will only make you stronger.

Let orin age for 2-3 months. The first few weeks it becomes very pungent in smell, but only if you have been

eating cooked foods, taking drugs or alcohol, animal or dairy products. When eating all raw foods and fruits, orin smells like the most amazing flowers or essential oil!

Any bad smells are easily remedied with a couple drops of essential oils (like lemon or rose) on top of the fabric (covering the orin jar) each day or as necessary. After about a month, orin loses its (ammonia) smell and turns neutral, dark, oxidizing and more potent.

Start aging and using orin today and regain your health.

Another good tip: Place a bucket or wide-open container (near the orin or simply in the same room) with hot water in it and drizzle a bit of bleach on top. Works like a

charm to get rid of the bad smell in the whole area/room for a few days!

Be sure to give the orin time to sit in the sun.

It's called "solarizing" and it is done by placing the open orin container under direct sunlight, at noon or during the strong hours of sunshine. An hour or two a day is enough. Up to ten days is good, enough to completely charge the orin with extra cosmic energy; from the cosmic body in the sky.

Remember that YOU are a sun in itself. Your soul emits energy, all the energy you need and all the energy you see in the universe. Your orin is already packed with that energy of your own soul. All these extra things/procedures are only a cherry on top. You can do just fine without them as well, but it is nevertheless another thing that you can do.

Boiling orin is never a good idea

While some recommend that, I prefer to let orin reduce its water content and get more concentrated in a natural way.

It takes longer but does not harm the nutrients, elements, stem cells in it with extreme temperatures. I don't think that's necessary to do to my living cells, so why would I do that to the living cells of my orin?

Reminder: the Orin aging process requires time and patience.

Using orin at any stage of its "aging or incubating" is still more potent than fresh orin. It will take being patient and willing to wait longer with each batch of stored orin, but you are worth it. You will be thankful you let orin age for longer periods.

Monica has been practicing Orin Therapy for over 22 years and started experimenting with drinking aged orin for 3 years ago. She realized that by rubbing it on the skin, it was also entering the body/blood stream and doing healing internally, so why not also drink it or use it in enemas and on open wounds. It would go right into the blood-stream through the open wound and in contact with the blood.

Not seeing a problem drinking orin, she has been doing

this for 3 years now. Sharing her experiences as a written document doesn't mean that everyone should follow what I say or do, it simply means that there is this other possibilities and everyone is free to choose the way they want to use their own free medicine.

Sediments found in orin

As orin is evolving, there is usually a build up of sediments at the bottom of the pee jar, in which particulates or crystals may appear. Metaphysical thinkers teach that this is really the renowned alchemical form of Ormus or white powder of Gold.

It has been explained that the white powdery formations that precipitated at the bottom of the container are white blood cells and also incapsulated within these white cells are stem cells. This is often the result of going off a raw vegan diet and eating cooked and proceed foods.

Cooked foods are notorious for causing acid conditions, dehydration and excess mucus (which causes obstruction, loss of vitality and inflammation).

Question: Does the aged stuff really have an odor?

Answer: It only smells bad, when the body and the diet are not cleaned properly and kept natural.

Mine took a long time to get to a beautiful clean state and it happened after several short and long orin fasts and months avoiding most cooked foods. I chose eating mostly fruits, everything 100% raw and natural, foods from mother nature and in their natural state.

Now my orin doesn't smell bad at all and it also doesn't acquire any bad or foul smell or taste afterwards when it's aging. I only need to make sure I am eating 100% fruitarian or raw vegan.

It's whenever I make an exception in my diet, that I observe my orin changing its smell and flavor. Cooked food, even a little amount of it, immediately will pollute my body and the orin reflects that, because it's the water running through this body as it shows whether it is clean or not.

After eating anything cooked (altered from its natural state) or foods that don't come from mother nature (from the plant kingdom), orin changes its smell and taste and becomes "filthy." That's because the body has become filthy.

But I know the best way to clean the body and make it return to its natural state.

It's precisely from drinking that "filthy"" orin. Filtering my own water again and again through this perfect filtration system cleans the body with all its organs.

My aged orin collected from a perfectly clean, natural and on a 100% raw fruitarian diet, no exceptions made, has the most wonderful smell. Really an amazing fragrance.

Reminds me of *the smell of newborn babies.*

Play it smart. It is simple, stay as close to living foods and fruit as possible. Build regular use in practice times of doing orin therapy. Orin is only as good as the person who uses it. *Monica Schütt*

17. Orin Bath

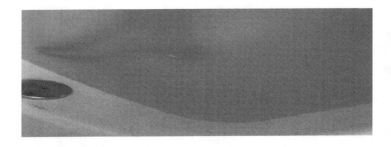

Collect a gallon or more of orin and prepare a bath with as hot of water that you can relax into comfortably. Be prepared to stay in the tub for 30 minutes. Using another jar of orin, rub the skin while in the orin bath.

Here's a simple way to knock out several protocols at once. Do this while filling up the bathtub. Be sure to bring some collected orin in a container or collect some on the spot.

Stand in the bath water as the tub is filling up.

Take the container of this water and start

drinking, gargling, swishing, pulling and swallowing.

Pour some over from either side of both of the eyes and into each ear. Do orin nose drinking either from a jar or palm of your hand, sniffing or snorting.

Thoroughly massage or rub orin into hair and scalp. Give yourself a good UT bodyrub all over the body as best that you can.

Be sure to apply orin to the navel and any skin conditions or wounds that could use healing.

Then soak and meditate in bath water with any left over orin either poured over the head and shoulders or any method you can imagine.

You can rinse off after taking a bath or leave it on and let it dry. That familiar pee smell evaporates quickly.

18. Skin conditions

The external application of orin to the skin allows hormones and nutrients to be re-absorbed by the body without being destroyed. Massaging with orin is therefore an important complementary component of orin therapy as it is directly absorbed into the tissue.

Orin is ideal for health. Since it detoxifies the body, strengthens the immune system, calms the nervous system, helps reduce weight by aiding digestion and elimination, reduces inflammation, cleanses the urinary tract, reduces a headache if you drink 1 to 8oz cup or more first thing in the morning or the onset of a headache and healing other conditions that you will soon know.

Orin is best known as a drink, but there are dozens of useful ways to use it in your daily life.

It is also one of the most effective natural ingredients for healthy skin and skin-related problems. The liver, btw, is the organ responsible for the health or lack of health of the skin.

Combining drinking pee with topical application restores both liver and skin health.

Urea (a substance found in orin) is one of the main reasons why it is often an ingredient in a variety of creams, peels, and lotions either made at home or bought in a store.

These can significantly improve the health of the skin, hair, teeth, nails and overall surface of the body.

Applying fresh orin on the skin before bedtime makes the face look healthier and younger. Using a cotton ball, washcloth or hand, apply wee on your face. And in the morning, you will notice incredible results. Soon you stop using face cream or any unnatural facial products.

Pee is a natural product that darkens, restores hair color, making it thicker and shinier. Many report that their hair looks better than when they were younger. Orin improves & nourishes the hair and scalp.

To do this, massage orin thoroughly into your hair. This trick will have a greater effect if you apply it to the hair shortly before going out into the intense sunlight. Leave it on as long as possible before washing hair again.

UT is a wonderful remedy for facial skin problems such as blackheads, dark spots, pigment spots, dried or cracked skin, acne and capillary bursts. Dabbing on orin with a soaked cotton ball, washcloth or hand heals skin problems.

Simply applying a little bit of your orin is enough. Apply directly to the affected areas and leave on the area for 10 minutes, then either wash with water or leave to dry. No residue or odor will remain.

Reminder: applying orin on the face or any skin surface still delivers its vital nutrients from the tissues to the bloodstream. Anywhere you apply orin on the body or drink it, delivers nutrients everywhere in the body.

In a cold atmosphere, the lips may dry out. To treat dried, infected or chapped lips, apply orin on the lips anytime or before bedtime to further increase hydration and heal. This will remove dead cells while it makes your lips soft and tender.

AUT eliminates blackheads & pimples. Teenagers love this.

Orin treats acne and blackheads on the face. Its antifungal and antibacterial characteristics help solve problems that disturb you, make you feel self-conscious or embarrassed.

Soak a cotton ball in the freshly collected Shivambhu and apply it to any skin surfaces with pimples.

Topical or external use of orin works wonders on insect or ant bites, wasp/hornet/bee stings, jellyfish stings, poison ivy or poison oak, burns, sunburn, eczema, bruises, dried or cracked skin, cuts, scratches or wounds.

Use your imagination and intuition when applying orin topically to treat any and all skin conditions.

Been in the sun too long? Not to worry.

Orin removes sunburn sting in 10 minutes as it quickly raises the alkaline pH (which is in chemistry, the values of the concentration of the hydrogen ion) of the skin and body.

Apply orin to any skin surfaces exposed to the sun after sunbathing. Within minutes the sting will be unnoticeable. A beautiful tan will be the reward for treating sunburn with orin.

Apply orin 2 more times during the next 24 hours to add nourishment to the skin and body. You be left with a lovely tan and no discomfort from any excess sun exposure.

19. Orin compresses and body wraps

Orin compresses and body wraps are effective in treating diseased body parts and internal organs, skin conditions and wounds.

These work miracles quickly when treating a third-degree burn. You may have to leave a compress on and keep it moist for three days to give the body a chance to grow a new layer of skin.

The open or swollen skin over the blister should be left alone, do not puncture it, since this protects the area serving as a temporary bandaid for the new layer of skin growing under the blister.

Refill the compress when it becomes dry, replace it and reapply.

20. Fresh orin rubbings

One method is to soak cotton balls or washcloth in orin and rub or dab on effected area(s). When treating an area that has been affected, get a soft latex disposable glove for hands), soft plastic type of shoe covers used by surgeons (for feet), plastic bags, shower cap (for brain and scalp), plastic wrap or the large leaf of a tree to cover to wrap the burned or affected area. This is done to keep oxygen away from the skin.

Oxygen is what causes the skin to blister and to feel painful.

Indication: General skincare, rashes, wounds and bites.

21. Homeopathic UT tinctures

Homeopathic remedies are based on un-related substances that coincidentally pro-duce a similar symptom picture.

These are great for chronically ill patients who have weakened systems and are going slow with their healing. It would serve them well as a first introductory step with UT.

A Homeopathic dose of orin affects the body in a similar way as being vaccinated against a certain disease, in which case, a small amount of poisonous substances is injected into a healthy body. Exception is that orin has no toxins, side effects or danger to our health.

This stimulates the immune system to manufacture antibodies (and thus defend the body), and could be called a homeopathic or isopathic effect. Isopathic remedies are made from the actual substances that cause allergic reactions or illnesses. For example, if you are allergic to cats, you could make a homeopathic remedy out of cat dander; if you're allergic to ragweed, diluted ragweed pollen would be an appropriate isopathic remedy.

This practice is different from standard homeopathic remedies, which are based on unrelated substances that produce a similar symptom picture.

The practice of drinking and massaging with orin allows the antibodies, greater access to the body, which stimulates the immune system.

Make a homeopathic tincture by putting a dropperful of orin in a 3-ounce bottle and fill it with distilled water. Apply one drop to a dropperful of tincture under the tongue, every four hours.

An alternative to a homeopathic tincture is to place 1-2 drops of fresh undilluted orin under tongue every four hours. Increase the dose every few days until client can handle 1 or more ounces. As they gain more strength, teach them how to trust their intuition to guide them to know when and how to increase the dosing.

The exciting or turning point happens in the mind when a client realizes that they have the power of their water to heal them. Many get very excited and motivated to get well at this point and move quickly into saturation dosing, looping and fasting.

With your guidance and encouragement along with their commitment to heal, another client will soon be free of disease, pain and anxiety.

22. Compress for hair, feet and hands

Fill silicon disposible gloves, shower cap, plastic leg cast protector or plastic bag, with fresh or evolving orin. Leave it on area for an hour, according to severity of burn, rash, bite, cut or sting. Do not apply creams or any other products on the skin.

If orin first aid is not available, forget the orin, immediately covering the burn area is the most important thing to do.

Refill your orin compress when it dries up. For a third-degree burn you may have to leave it on for three days to give the body a chance to grow a new layer of skin.

Enjoy watching these unique protocols for healing conditions of the brain, hands and feet.

facebook.com/brothersage/
videos/10156468190221529/

Throughout history Sages have been well aware of the hormonal effects of orin. They state that if a person is unable to urinate, the orin from somebody of the same sex is acceptable but not from somebody of the other sex.

It has been a long held belief that female orin contains greater amounts of female hormones such as estrogen and if ingested over a long period of time by a man, this may have a feminizing effect. The opposite was also believed to be true for a woman who ingests male orin which contains extra testosterone.

Despite this theory or superstition, many report that when Orin Therapy is needed to restore health, orin from either gender, will do just fine. Shivambhu is known as a universal panacea for a reason.

For patients who are unable to keep down fluids or urinate, obtain orin from another person other than the patient to give it to a person who is sick. The "preferred" donor is a vegan, non-smoker who does not take drugs or drink alcohol.

This method of using the orin of a donor works well because orin is neither gender, age or race specific.

Some UT therapists, like Doc Mike Witort* of Chicago with over 20 years of UT experience, proved this point to his seriously ill clients by drinking their orin (both genders) even from those diagnosed wth cancer, diabetes or a virus. They are all getting great results.

Rub or massage the whole body or the affected area with orin. Leave it on or rinse it off with cool water after 15 minutes. Avoid use of soap.

Note: For topical use, applying orin that is at least 8 days old is better than two day old orin. Save it in a glass jar with a good cover, in a cool and dark place.

Obtain orin immediately after intercourse and apply it to the genitals and related area. Girls should apply a douche with fresh orin. Leave the orin on the skin for at least 10 minutes.

Breathe in vapors of orin (either from the palm of a hand, mister, spray top bottle or nebulizer (diffusor) 2 to 3 times a day until the healing crisis occurs.

Change or complement your diet with raw foods. A more simpler and for some, challenging way of eating, is the fruitarian lifestyle.

23. Orin Deodorant

As one improves the quality of their diet and continues with UT, you will begin to have more pleasant smelling sweat or perspiration. This lets you stop using a commercial under arm deodorant.

As *a deodorant*, dab some orin in the places where you usually roll on an antiperspirant. The result will be remarkable. One will not smell from sweat. Rub on hairy chests and feet for a clean and fresh tropical fragrance.

Practicing UT protocols daily, especially with the addition of saturation dosing, builds a strong body as it quickens the healing.

24. Orin by the bedside

Keep a small size jar of orin on a nightstand next to your bed. Many leave the jar open without a lid all night for air purification, deep sleep and improved breathing. This orin can be useful to quench a thirst in the night or to put in the navel as a way to return to a deeper sleep or on the legs to heal leg cramps or a charley horse.

Get used to your friends commenting on how you look glowing, ageless and more relaxed.

Drinking one's pee can wake you up!

Orin Juice: 100% pure therapeutic grade ultra filtered golden blood plasma water is what does a body good.

To overcome doubts about the power of Orin by clients, carefully read the following.

Practical suggestions for those starting Shivambhu. Tread gently by Manjushree Abhinav*

1) Soak your feet in fresh Shivambhu (pee standing in a small tub/ bucket), for five to ten minutes. See how soft your feet feel, how fresh you feel. Get familiar with your living waters.

2) Soak your feet in cooled Shivambhu. This is the ultimate luxury for those living in hot countries. This draws the toxins out of your feet plus gives you a natural pedicure.

3) Collect the first pee of the morning, mid-stream, mix in half with water. To begin with, drink only a couple of spoons of this mix, let your body slowly get accustomed to the taste of Shivambhu. And if you start slow, the detoxifying symptoms will probably not be too intense. Be prepared for detox symptoms, like lose stools, headache, slight fever or nausea, in the first week or two of starting the practice.

This won't last long, and if you accept it without complaint or fear, it will go sooner.

4) The second pee in the morning should be used for 5 things: wash face and neck, fill up an eye cup and wash eyes, add a little rock salt and clean the teeth with fingers (gum massage) and then the toothbrush, orin pulling, and pour some in the belly button. I have stopped using moisturiser, toothpaste and soap for the face. In case of a cough, warm up some Shivambhu (do not boil, only slightly warm), add rock salt, like himalayan crystal salt and gargle.

5) Collect the pee during the day and store it in glass bottles, secure with a clean cotton cloth and rubber bands. Keep this glass bottle near a window or in the open, so that sunlight falls on it. After 15 to 21 days, the Shivambhu will lose its intense smell and darken.

This can be used for self body massage, better known as a pee bath. Take some of it in a wide mouthed cup, pour some fresh Shivambhu to add volume, dip your hands in it and rub, rub, rub the whole body with it till it absorbs all of it and turns almost dry, meaning it is absorbed back in the body through the skin.

Give special attention to painful areas. You can use a cloth for the back. Wash off with water (do not use soap or shampoo), and you'll be surprised to find that there is no smell, on the contrary, a very clean, sublime feeling.

Like a baby, loved and cherished. Let go of all your angst, and relax in the sheer abundance of this self love.

(Regular pee baths will make you as strong as an elephant —Dr. Sarang Patil)

6) When you are ready, start drinking more and more Shivambhu, and allow your body to naturally change the diet toward eating more fruits, salads, less sugar, less fried stuff, and introduce weekly fasts wherein you drink all the Shivambhu you pass during the day along with water.

This is called Amaroli kriya, orin fast or looping. You won't feel hungry, as Shivambhu makes sure you get all the required nutrients you need. You can also use looping during intermittent fasting, like skipping breakfast. Great for losing weight.

7) Generally, two glasses of Shivambhu, one

in the morning and one in the evening are good enough. Wait for a couple of hours after food before having it. And fifteen minutes of waiting after having Shivambhu, before you eat/drink. Plain water can be had any time.

8) If Shivambhu is too strong an experience for you, try homeopathic doses of it. It is very effective as an emergency medicine, for such conditions like fever, panic attack, backaches.

9) Avoid using chemically strong things like hair colour, perfumes, powder, lipstick, make up, face creams, bleaches, or scrubs. Go herbal. Better still, go minimal. Shivambhu is the god-given provider. Regular use of it will eliminate the need for all these.

10) Those of you who are using tobacco, marijuana, or alcohol, and have thought of giving up the habit, simply start drinking your living water, the Shivambhu will guide you to gradually to stop the self abuse without effort, because this practice holistically guides you toward self love.

11) In case of constipation, or digestion problems, aged shivambhu enemas are amazing and can be a lifesaver. Enemas need not be a

big project. A small rubber bulb / a syringe filled with matured Shivambhu can be used.

12) Drinking Shivambhu through the nose is good for the brain. It clears brain fog and brings a twinkle to the eyes.

—Manjushree Abhinav*

Nourishes the nails

To strengthen, nourish, refresh and brighten the color of your nails, soak them in orin for 10-15 minutes. Then, brush the nails. In the end, rinse your nails in water or orin. You will be pleasantly surprised by the results.

Enemas and fasting greatly improve the cleansing and purification of the body, mind and spirit.

1. Choosing the right container(s).

The Shiva Khalpa (from the Damar Tantra scriptures) recommends the use of pots made of gold, silver, copper, brass, iron, glass, earth or clay, bamboo, bones, leather or a bowl made of plantain leaves as the ideal containers to use to store orin.

2. **What to use as a cover** – cheese cloth, soft material or nylon stocking can stretch to cover any size jar. Covering an orin jar is optional. As orin is ultra antiseptic and antibacterial, you can simply screw on jar lid and leave orin alone to evolve gracefully.

3. **Labeling the storage date** lets us measure the "age," strength and any unusual changes in the evolving orin.

Since there is no special formula to determine when orin will reach its "nutritional peak." Trust intuition and personal experience as the best indicator of the strength of the evolving orin. Orin users have reported storing evolving orin for 9 or more years.

By its nature, Shivambhu is self-purifying and always evolving. Where can you find anything like Shivambhu in nature? Perhaps its what a salamander uses to regrow a tail.

It is a personal choice whether to cover the orin jar with a material or screw on lid. As the world's most renowned antiviral, antibacterial, antiseptic, antifungal and anti pathogenic substance, no toxic bacteria can compromise or grow in orin.

Rest, Rest, Rest

After you are healed and in good health, continuing the daily practice with UT protocols and a good diet will be your best insurance for a long and healthy life. Never allow yourself to become regularly exhausted or overtired. Consistent proper rest is crucial to health. Once you have recovered from a major illness or from pushing yourself too hard to accomplish anything, stay vigilant and mindful in getting abundant rest and relaxation.

Chapter 8
Offering suggestions without prescribing or diagnosing

You and a client can only succeed when you are of service, when you guide, mentor and are not a personality, ego, or identity who is seeking praise or has an attachment to the outcome. Orin Therapy teachers never make promises of healing with a client. The ultimate responsibility in healing with UT rests in the mind of the client. Give your best and expect the best.

One of the most interesting pieces of information on orin that I came across was the fact that the amniotic fluid that surrounds human infants in the womb is primarily orin. The infant "breathes in" orin-filled amniotic fluid continually.

Without this fluid, the lungs don't develop.

Doctors believe that the softness of a baby's skin and the ability of in-utero infants to heal quickly without scarring after pre-birth surgery is due to the therapeutic properties of the orin-filled amniotic fluid.

UT works for some and not for everyone. Why?

Healing is more complex than just drinking orin. Improving the diet, fasting, cleansing, right thinking or attitude, healthy emotions and spiritual or self-love practices will boost Shivambhu benefits.

Understand?

People who are miserable inside or self-destructive have much more work to do then do grateful, joyous people.

Motived people do really well with Orin Therapy.

A well-trained or intuitively sensitive UT therapist will make inquiries into all areas of the client's life and design a well-rounded program that accelerates, deepens and brings results. Detailed questioning is more thorough than just advising clients to do UT protocols and wish them well.

Taking the time to do follow ups brings confidence and reassurance to the client as you are working as a team to change, save and improve a life.

Studying and knowing the basics of the nutritional profile of orin, builds one's skill in making inquiries, addressing concerns and offering UT protocol suggestions.

For example, working with clients who are stressed, exhausted or have low energy, you may wish to remind them that orin contains nutrients, such as melatonin, serotonin, magnesium, DHEA, dopamine, L-theanine, Phenylalanine, niacin, tryptophan, oxytocin and B-complex that are well known to support the function of the adrenals, glands, nervous system and brain.

Knowing this about orin, of course, is optional and does not affect the outcome or benefits of AUT for a client. It just adds more credibility and respect from clients who value this type of information. If you feel that in addition to their "health condition," they are anxious with concerns about life, your sensitivity and intuition will guide and assist you to help clients more during a session.

Shivambhu is love

In this Manual there are articles from UT educators, Researchers and teachers on Shivambhu self-healing practices. These are written to help you to design "perfect" treatment suggestions.

In the popular Shivambhu Hut, social media network*, you can read UT articles and watch related videos, as well as contribute content that is being enjoyed by the members of the growing water family at the Hut. To get a free membership visit the Shivambhu Hut entrance portal at https://shivambhu.org/shivambhu-hut.

To avoid making claims and keep yourself from any legal matters, always remember that you are not a licensed medical professional who can diagnose and prescribe medications.

Study general treatment suggestions.

Stay on the safe side and only guide them along their Shivambhu journey.

Remind them that the body heals itself when given the proper nutrients and those nutrients are absorbed. Mention that their body's innate intelligence custom manufactures the perfect elixir for their specific needs every time. This is most important to know.

Chapter 9
General treatment suggestions

This list contains some of the most commonly labeled dis-eases and UT protocol suggestions from the classic book, Golden Fountain: The complete book on Urine Therapy by Coen van der Kroon. *

The beneficial effects of practicing Orin Therapy may vary according to a client's diet, lifestyle, state of mind and way of being and commitment. Benefits will range from some relief to total healing, and in general one must realize that healing is always dependent upon many co-factors.

In this chapter of the Manual you will find the precise methods in detail.

As was mentioned in the discussion in the Whole Body (Body/Mind) healing chapter: All four pillars of health must be in balance to achieve optimum health. These areas include mental, emotional, physical and self-love or "spiritual."

There are no strict guidelines or rules for UT. Starting from a general, basic treatment, everyone must find the application of UT which is most appropriate for their needs and, similarly, which other types of treatment should be combined with UT for the best results.

Generally, in cases of chronic or serious diseases, it is useful to do an orin fast with distilled water, foot soaks, navel soaks, orin enemas and have regular orin massages. This is referred to as an "intensive treatment." In most cases, even when relatively healthy, this intense form of UT is highly cleansing and health giving.

Whenever massage is mentioned in these treatment suggestions, you get to decide whether to use evolving (maturing or culturing) orin (see chapter "Evolving (Aged) orin" vs. Fresh Orin) or fresh orin.

Evolving orin has more potency

The term "massage" generally means the gentle rubbing of orin into the skin or applying it to the affected parts.

Conditions General Treatment Suggestions

Visit Chapter 7 to learn any protocols listed here next to the condition.

Acne—wash face with orin, orin fast, drinking

Aging—several glasses a day as a general tonic, nose drinking, massage

AIDS—saturation doses, drinking, massage, enemas

Allergies—enemas, naval soak, injections, fasting

Amoebas—(virus, pathogens, bacteria) drinking, fasting, enemas **Anemia** drinking, bath, massage, dietary changes

Apathy—drinking, nose drinking, foot soak, massage

Appendicitis—(all inflammation) drinking, nose drinking, compresses

Arthritis—drinking, nose drinking, compresses

Asthma—(all lung issues) saturation doses, drinking, dietary changes

Athletes Foot/Foot fungus—saturation doses, drinking, massage, enemas

Atrophy—drinking, nose drinking, massage

Backache—massage, drinking, compresses, foot soak

Bites—drinking, massage, compresses, rubbings

Bladder problems—drinking, compresses, nose drinking

Blisters—compress, rubbing, drinking

Blood pressure (low)—drinking, dietary changes, massage, foot soaks

Blood pressure (high)—drinking (moderately), dietary changes

Blood vessels (constriction of)—drinking, nose drinking, bath

Boils—Rubbing on boils, drinking, compresses

Bowel movement (constipation, colitis, IBS)—drinking, enemas, naval soak, massage, foot soak

Brain injury or related diseases—drinking, compresses to the head, scalp massage

Bronchitis—saturation doses, drinking, nose drinking, injection, compress, massage

Burns—Massage, compress, drinking and bath

Cancer (all Cancer)—saturation dosing, drinking, enemas, foot soaks, massage

Candidiasis—drinking, enemas, naval soak, fasting

Cataracts—(all eye problems) eye wash, drinking, nose drinking and foot soaks

Cold (cough)—drinking, gargling, pulling, nose drinking

Cysts—massage, compresses

Dandruff—massage hair and scalp, drinking

Depression—drinking, nose drinking, foot soaks, massage, naval soak

Diabetes—drinking, dietary changes, massage, foot soak

Diarrhea—drinking, fasting, enemas

Digestion issues—drinking, fasting, foot soak, naval soak and massage

Dizziness—drinking, compresses to the head, naval soak, nose drinking

Ear problems—ear rinses, drinking, foot soaks, nose drinking

Eczema—massage, compresses, injection

Energy (fatigue)—drinking, drinking aged orin, sniffing or nose drinking

Fever (migraine, headache)—drinking, massage, fasting, compresses, nose drinking

Fungus—massage, compress, drinking, enemas

Gall Bladder issues—drinking, fasting, dietary changes, foot soak

Gum (all mouth) conditions—gargling, swishing, pulling, drinking, looping

Hair Loss—massage hair with fresh or aged orin, drinking

Heart conditions—drinking, looping, body massage, foot soaks, naval soak, nose drinking

Hepatitis—drinking, fasting, compresses to the liver, foot soak

Insect bites, stings—put on affected areas, compress, drinking

Itching—put on affected areas, massage

Kidney problems—drinking, dietary change, compress on kidney areas

Lyme—drinking, fasting, enemas, foot soak

MS—drinking, fasting, enemas

Menopause—drinking, foot soaks including the ankles

Obesity—drinking, fasting, dietary changes, enemas, foot & naval soaks

Parasites—drinking, fasting, enemas

Prostate disorders—drinking, fasting, enemas, massage, compress on affected area

Scars (skin conditions)—compresses, massage, drinking

Sciatica—drinking, massage, compresses

Sexual potency or drive—drinking, nose drinking, navel soak, massage genitals

Shock—drinking own water or someone else's if needed, Navel & foot soaks

Spasms—drinking, massage, naval soak

Stomach problems—drinking, massage, navel soaks

Stress—drinking, nose drinking, foot soaks, massage

Sunburn—apply to affected areas, bath &

drinking

Tinnitus—ear rinses, nose drinking, drinking, yoga

Tooth issues—gargling, swishing, pulling, looping

Ulcer—massage, drinking, compress, foot & navel soaks

UTI—drinking, foot soak

Vaginal problems—douche, washing area, drinking, massage

Warts—apply to affected areas, drinking

Wounds—apply to affected areas, drinking

Chapter 10
Designing UT protocols and wellness practices For a client to bring radiant health

Making inquiries or probing into the lives of a client determines the direction of the session. This information compiled from the discussion helps in designing general treatment suggestions and a program that includes all aspects of well-being.

Inquiry helps you understand a holistic overview of their life as as way of building protocols, practices and a program that brings the results they came to you to achieve.

Just telling them to drink their water and try UT protocols and sending them away to figure it all out is not only a disservice to a client, but they will have a much harder journey when only approaching health from only the physical or material form.

Here are some sample questions for new clients to contemplate and answer.

What motivated you to start practicing UT? A book, person or illness? Who or what was your influence?

What went through mind when you were considering actually drinking your pee?

Can you recall any defining moments that stand out that inspired your decision?

What mental obstacles, if any, did you have to overcome to take the first drink?

Was it easy or difficult for you to do this? Did you have to overcome a gag reflex or feelings of disgust?

What UT protocols are you currently practicing and which do you use everyday?

Have you tried a variety of the UT protocols? Which are your favorites and why?

What did you study or what are you studying to further your UT education?

Would you say that you are passionate and outspoken about Shivambhu?

Are you serious about telling others about your UT discovery and personal success with UT?

How has daily UT practices affected your life?

Do you think that you will ever consider that you might stop doing this practice?

Can you explain the transition that people go through in order to get the most from practicing UT, ie: diet (food choices), lifestyle, mental changes or beliefs about oneself.

What advice would you give to newbies about taking that important first sip?

Chapter 11
Clearing the mind of all negative associations, beliefs or ideas about UT, including suggestions, theories, and myths taught to you, especially by the medical industry

Learning a client's beliefs about orin and if they ever considered drinking their pee, gives you a clearer picture of which direction to take the conversation and initial consultation.

Beatrice Barnett in her book, *The Miracles of Urine Therapy*, offers a good approach to handling aversions to drinking orin. Throughout the civilized world, blood and blood products are being used in the medical world without evoking the repugnance associated with orin.

We use prepackaged cells, blood plasma, white blood cells and countless other blood components. Orin is nothing other than a blood plasma product.

Babies are being breast-fed and we easily accept this along with the common practice of eating dairy products.

Yet we cannot imagine drinking orin. Fresh orin contains the same substances as those found in the blood. If you think about it, orin is ultra filtered blood plasma water.

Pee was part of your blood just minutes before and flowed elsewhere through your body, possibly through your tongue.

Since orin is not poisonous or disgusting while in the body, why is it considered so repulsive as piss?

Overcoming objections in a sensitive and compassionate manner is crucial to a successful UT session. Anyone who criticizes or challenges you about Orin Therapy (whether someone in person or someone who calls in to a radio show while you are being interviewed, known as a heckler or troll) is someone who never did their research and is repeating what they have been taught about orin.

This way you never take their words, energy or emotions personally and you can hold your ground while confidently responding to them.

Bring it on, baby!!!!

Some of the concerns or mental obstacles that have been overcome about drinking orin, has included:

I've always thought it was a waste product.

Why would anyone wanna drink their pee?

They are secretly wondering if you are a trusted or credible source?

They seem to be waiting for guidance from the inner voice, to decide about working with you.

These are the pillars of health and wellbeing: Mental. Emotional. Physical. Self Love (spiritual).

It is to your advantage, dear readers, to take this teaching to heart and design a personal daily program of practices for you first.

After being a product of discipline, you will know how to assist your clients in finding their way.

1.What will they (parents, siblings, children or partner) think of me if I become a pee drinker?

Remind the client that what they think about themselves matters most. What others think about you is none of your business. Your work will include acknowledging and giving them recognition, empowering them and reminding them the truth about themselves.

I am going to feel embarrassed and think that others are criticizing me.

Once again, give client reassurance that they are ok just as they are right now.

Are you insane or in a cult?

Trust issue. Give reassurance.

Is it safe?

Trust issue. Give reassurance. I have been drinking my pee for many years and I feel greater everyday. 30 million people worldwide are alive and well because they drink their wee every day.

Does that tell you anything?

Q: Is orin really sterile or full of germs?

A: Being made in the ultimate sterile environment without any contact from outside the body, your water is being made in ultra-sterile laboratory conditions. It is always designed exactly to meet your most current bodily needs, stored in a sterile container (the bladder) and then signals you by using pressure that your elixir is ready.

Orin is absolutely sterile and most of the orin that your body produces goes back into the bloodstream anyway.

Q: Why does orin smell sometimes?

A: After awhile the uric acid in orin changes into ammonia, and only then does it start to smell. However, the smell evaporates completely after the orin is absorbed into the skin, or any organic surface.

Got any testimonials* or research† that might convince me?

Yes there are 1,000's to show you. What will it take for you to trust my word and get stated?

Wow! Was it hard for you to take that first drink?

I was 40 at the time and had experimented with just about everything imaginable.

Considering all the many methods of healing that I have tried as a way to become healthy, drinking my pee was not much of a leap.

What really convinced me to go for that first sip and drink was the writings of Coen van der Kroon (The Golden Fountain, my UT Bible*) and Leonard Orr (The Secrets of Youthing). It was the reminder by Leonard, a devotee of Babaji (known by many as Lord Shiva) that spoke to me.

Well, since Shiva sent Leonard to deliver the Shivambhu message to me, of course I said yes.

What has it done for you?

It has healed the intestines, vision improved, hearing sharpened and calmed this restless mind. Keeping the discipline of using of UT protocols everyday for 26 years continues to bring me a clear / calm mind, balanced emotions and boundless energy all day.

"I have always thought that it was a waste product. It's what I always heard about piss."

Where did you get that idea? What made you think that was true? Perhaps the medical system made it all up to hide the knowledge of Shivambhu from us.

Why would anyone want to drink his or her pee?

When I am done explaining the truth about orin and have answered all of your questions, you will be convinced.

Only when your motivation or "Why" is strong enough to take action to get well, will you hear and understand why millions are healthier and happier because they made the choice to begin and practice AUT every day.

Trust me. You will pee glad you did.

Why should I trust you or take your word for it that it is safe & healthy for me to drink my pee?

Do I appear sane and sincere that AUT is the real deal?

Check in with yourself now and see how you feel about AUT and if you are ready to go for it.

By planting this one idea in their mind, concerns start to wash away as they sense your certainty and sincerity about AUT's potential to help restore their health.

What if we are right and *urine really is* perfect medicine and the medical system got it wrong?

Okay, now you got my attention.
How do I start?

Reminder: you and you client can only succeed as long as you take the position of a servant, guide, mentor and not a personality, ego or identity that is seeking to prove anything.

1) Offer a personal AUT story as confirmation or validation that you got results (proving to them that you are not a snake oil sales person, are sincere and do walk your talk). You can also offer the stories of others ("third party") to satisfy their need for testimonials.

Teach what AUT has done for others. Learn how UT teachers are designing general suggestions (chapter 9 on general treatment suggestions).

2) Teach basic UT 101. Keep it simple. Avoid talking over their head no matter how much they appear to know. Get in the habit of thinking that you are speaking to a fifth grader and you'll be effectively communicating with most people.

There is of course, not much you can do with skeptics or closed minds. Yet, you have planted a seed, which may take root and grow someday.

Those that are serious about saving their lives and healing themselves will be listening and will take your advice.

Teach the joy of drinking one's own water (orin) and all AUT protocols. Clients will guide you in taking the next step and dive deeper into the AUT Lifestyle.

When a doctor claims that any disease is incurable, what they really means is that their limited education and profession does not include self-healing and cannot help you.

Doctors do not promote AUT either because *they don't know about it or **they do know about it*** and will lose their reputation, license and practice if they tell the truth.

The word "incurable" really means "in-cure-able." Meaning that from *within, **we are cure able***. Understanding this word in a new way reveals that healing is an inside job. Orin is *the* "cure-able" miracle drink that is already available to you right now.

3) Keep in mind that practicing AUT every day is a lifestyle choice, which requires a strong connection to Shivambhu, your body, daily discipline and utmost Faith.

4) When a client is ready to learn about AUT and how to present it to others, **that's when their Shivambhu Journey really begins**.

 Use your own free personal curative to re-claim health and well-being without any expense. The only costs are containers with lids or soft cloth material with rubber band to store the orin, 1-2 eye cups, enema bag with tube, clamp all related supplies, neti pot, cotton balls, wash cloth, tongue cleaner (free from a dentist), 1-3 oz size glass dropper bottle with dropper, 2 gallon "Tupperware" tub,

Q-tips, an 8-ounce cup and a good imagination.

On being a trusted source for clients

Establishing trust and a connection with students and clients is achieved from the skills and expertise you keep developing as an Orin Therapy professional. Relationships with clients get easier as you bring a clear state of mind, calm energy, sensitivity and presence into every meeting with them.

Relationship-building develops organically into mutual trust and admiration.

Remember: it is not up to you to make any decisions, set rules or boundaries for your clients. As with any form of therapy, you are the facilitator (guide) of every session or consultation. Despite how a client may perceive you, you are not to presume any role as a healer, saviour or authority for them.

The responsibility for healing and wellbeing is always up to the client. "A mere shift of perception is all that is required to heal oneself" A Course in Miracles

Your work is to teach information that will lead a client to learn their own unique way on this path. This empowers them to become motivated and self-disciplined in restoring their health and well-being.

When a client is excited or inspired by "WHY" they are drinking pee and using UT protcols daily, then their commitment and success is assured.

You just "did your job" and made a best friend for life.

Urine Therapy Shortcut
Teaching Method * (https://www.
facebook.com/brothersage/
videos/10157125188186529/)

Lead with this question: Do you think urine can be beneficial to one's own health? This gets them thinking about it, and "no" is the usual answer. "I was always taught that piss is toxic, so my reaction has always been that it is disgusting and smells, well, like pee."

This is when you remind them of situations in which urine is commonly used. Peeing on your feet for athlete's foot/fungus or smelling feet. Soldiers are taught in the Army Survival Manual to drink pee for survival, if stranded on a desert, or out in the ocean. To this they respond with Yes, but that is the only time I would drink it, would be to save my life. OK, now we agree it can save your life! Bingo. Your door of opportunity just presented itself. How can something that is toxic or a waste material save your life? Their mind just made room to hear what you have to say about Urine Therapy. Breathe.

Relax and in your own way, briefly tell them what you know about Urine Therapy.

This is the point where the topic can be discussed more openly, without you being labelled as a complete idiot or someone that is crazy. I always love to throw in the line " You know you have drank your own urine before." And they all reply they haven't, lol.

Then I go into the "Baby in the Womb - Amniotic Fluid is Pee" teaching.

Where the conversation goes from this point is up to you.

Call Brother Sage if you need a backup on your team.

Don't Worry Pee HapPee.

It is the Shivambhu High that has created millions of Shivambhu devotees across earth who are keeping up this practice every day as their secret health program.

Orin Therapy can be easily explained. No

complicated laboratory tests are required, no intricate scientific explanations are necessary and no diagnosis is needed.

Remind clients that there are no risks, danger or negative side effects to worry about other than possible cleansing and healing reactions. You will be asked to be willing to adjust many of your activities and considerations so you can focus your attention on the study and practice of AUT.

Once a person starts drinking pee and including topical protocols, clients see results rather quickly and make the commitment to stay with AUT.

There have been many scientific reports that validate this theory. Many people with serious conditions are improving considerably in a week up to a month, on average.

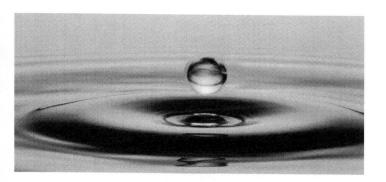

Chapter 12
Surveying a client

Before doing an inquiry, study and learn questions, like these, that you'll be using in interviews with clients.

Why pee? Why would you want to drink pee?

What do you think is the truth about orin?

What or who was your influence?

Can you recall any defining moments that may stand out that inspired your decision?

What mental obstacles, if any, did you have to overcome to take that first drink?

Are you ready to make a commitment to

practice UT?

For a newbie: Did you experience a "gag reflex" at any time during your first drink of pee?

Was it easy or difficult for you to do this?

Do you have the courage to tell others about UT?

Besides drinking orin, are you open to trying any of the protocols and have your own direct experience, so you will really know what Shivambhu can do for you?

Have you tried any of the topical UT protocols? Which are your favorites and why?

Where did you get your UT education?

Are you serious about telling others about your UT discovery and personal success with the protocols?

How has keeping up your daily UT practices affected your wellbeing or life?

Do you think that you will ever consider stopping this practice?

Can you explain the changes that you are going through that is giving you the best results with UT, i.e. diet (food choices), lifestyle, way of being or mindset?

What advice would you give to UT newbies about taking that important first step?

Chapter 13
Preparing for a UT session

How a teacher prepares for a UT session is just as important for the teacher as it is for the client. With the general understanding of Orin Therapy from studying this Manual and other UT resources, personal experience and teaching AUT, *you are already to be an AUT teacher.*

The work begins when you are present (really listening) with a client, following your intuition and knowing and/or trusting that the session will be perfect in every way.

You no longer have to think about what to say or what to do because Source is directing you.

In this chapter, we explore the use of the breath, meditation, centering and trusting ones inner knowing or guidance before starting a session with a client.

Being calm, centered and present gives you deeper insight into a client's emotions that arises from unconscious beliefs, programming and mental patterns that are at the core of their "health problems."

All names and labels of what the medical system calls dis-ease or illness is based on a diagnosis or theories, which comes from their medical education and is merely a suggestion. According to don Miguel Ruiz, author of *The Four Agreements*, modern medical practices are a form of black magic or hypnotic suggestion.

Being present with clients causes insights and guidance to go much deeper, be more accurate and bring more benefits. We are not only facilitating the session, we are guiding the client in using the mind to change beliefs about themselves and their life.

We are bringing hope, courage, strength and motivation to every client. Mastering the daily practice of AUT, teaches you how to teach others how to master the discipline needed to heal and accomplish anything.

Using your own breath and meditation practices or rituals before or during a session, sets the stage or energy for you to get the most out of each session.

It is a good idea to set aside time to lay or sit down and practice doing a minimum of 30 conscious connected breathing cycles every day. Spend at least 20 - 30 minutes meditating, taking a walk quietly in Nature and being still and silent in mind, energy and body.

Breathe. *Let go of all that matter that doesn't really matter.*

It is very important in counseling or coaching clients to teach them these yogic practices. This supports them through all their adjustment period they will be facing along their UT journey.

Teaching others to practice daily conscious connected breathing creates calm and joyous humans who (by the nature of their mindfulness to their breath while in the presence of others) are spreading conscious breath work to countless numbers of people during their life journey.

Other centering practices may include Tai Chi, Qi Gong, chanting, meditation, laughing, dancing, doing art projects like sculpting and painting or drawing pictures.

Every student may get inspired to either share Orin Therapy with others or become a UT teacher some day. Always look at the "big picture of UT for all humanity" and how every person is affecting evolution for future generations.

Chapter 14
Looking into an
Orin Therapy session

Remember that clients are seeking you for guidance, counsel and to be on their healing team. That is all that we really need to know.

Invite client to breathe, shuffle bare feet on the floor or carpet and clear the mind of chatter so they are present with you and ready to get started.

Returning a client's mind to balance, moves their thoughts away fom conflict, hopelessness and fear to a mind open to the possibility of being healthy, happy and free again.

At this point, you can begin inquiries or just listen.

Many bring their anxieties and concerns

about their "illness or condition" to the session of conversation, so keep reminding them to breathe.

You are building a relationship with every client. Your role is multifaceted and you can appear to play many roles for them. As you move through a session, discovering as much as you can about their diet, lifestyle, self-care and mindset, you are listening for clues to reveal the true cause of their "illness."

You'll get to know them as well as they know themselves by focusing on their words, thinking and energy. Find out why they chose UT as their method for self healing.

Since they chose you to coach them for their healing, they trust you.

It is this trust of you that will keep their mind open to your questioning, guidance and suggestions. Breathe. Remind them often to take deep breaths. Great. "Let's get started."
During the inquiry stage of the consultation, the questions you will ask are in no particular order.

What are your health concerns?

What do you normally eat?

What size are the proportions?

How many meals a day?

How often?

How late?

Do you chew thoroughly, like 20 times?

How early do you eat?

What did you eat today?

What do you do to relax? What time do you go to sleep at night? When do you get up in the morning?

How do you quiet your mind?

What if any are some of the spiritual practices like meditation, chanting, yoga, silence?

 Do you practice intermittent or regular fasting? Enemas?

As you are gathering information, you are also listening to their choice of words, descriptions and emotions they express behind their words.

You get better each time that you guide or facilitate a session at "reading" a client and getting insights that are beyond your education or intelligence.

Your intuition will show you what they have been believing about themselves, their body and their relationships. You can choose to help them process and clear their negative and limiting believes. Or lovingly and sensitively listen deeply and offer treatment suggestions, dietary and lifestyle choices, and teach them how to enjoy a life worth living.

Giving them positive affirmations will help them to raise the quality of their thoughts about themselves and their life. Never underestimate the power of affirmations that could bring about shifts of perception that could be heard, felt and integrated at any time during the session.

Ask the client if they are open to a quantum healing or to the possibility of healing everything in one or more sessions.

Your intention and attention to details will take the basic consultation, into becoming a transformational and life changing session for both of you.

Giving assignments, practices and resources helps build a solid foundation to start and continue their UT practices for life.

A good way for you both to stay present and "on the same page" is the use of audio or video recordings of every session. Remember to suggest recording the session as a way to give them the chance to give their permission or to refuse.

This will avoid any distractions and allow the conversation to flow much easier.

A teacher or therapist will naturally be taking notes or key points of what is being said. We will also be writing down insights the guidance (from your intuition or "inner voice") as best that they can and still keep up with the conversation.

Remind them that you will be sending them a link or a copy of the recording of the session, which held as confidential. Clients may, on occasion, give you permission to transcribe any non-personal information that can be used toward any new training material.

Use sensitivity and discernment if or when that you feel that it is appropriate to challenge them in anyway or call them out on their beliefs, issues, behaviors or diet.

Simply ask permission and then you can go for it.

Near the close of each session let them know that their time is almost up and ask if they have any closing remarks before we schedule our next session.

Did you enjoy our session?

If you get stuck, confused, scared or concerned about your UT practices, changes occurring in the body or if you're doing UT correctly, let me know. A UT therapist often makes good friends with a client. This lets them know that they can reach out to you for support or feedback between sessions.

Keep up your disciplines and so will your clients.

Roll up your sleeves, guys. It's time to be of service and give the client your best work. As you continue studying UT, practice the following:

(1) Calm the mind and become aware of the Presence (some call Love, the Light, Source energy, God or Life). Now you are ready to begin a session. Breathe. Let go and relax.

It's a conversation that matters with you as their guide and loving friend.

(2) Listening, paying close attention to what is being said and what is not being said, lets you hear what is just beneath their words.

(3) Compassion is the art of feeling what they are feeling as well as what you are feeling or "picking up" from their words, body language and energy. Use of compassion will bring comfort and safety to a client.

Then you can take the first step. The stages or steps will be discussed in more detail later in this chapter. These include (1) Making the internal shift to unlearn what you have been told about orin.

(2) Having the "discovery or ahha or breakthrough" known as the "adjustment period" (this is often felt as if one is dying or breaking apart but is in truth a mere shift of perception disguised as a breakthrough) or "integration."

(3) Finally after the integration stage, the client knows they are home by a feeling of wholeness, peace or home to the real or authentic self.

Drop into your calm center; be sensitive, compassionate and present. You are about to give 100% of your abilities (talent, time, training, education, experiences, energy, sensitivity, compassion and love) to the client in the session.

Although most UT sessions average 60–75 minutes in duration, you and the client will feel or know when the session is ending or chooses to continue until it is complete.

Grab a notebook and pen before session begins. You will be writing down as much of what the client is saying as possible. These notes will give you clues "in real time" by

How the client is describing, feeling and thinking about their health, body, their life and themselves.

Your ability to listen *to what is **not** being said* is just as important as *to what **is** being said* by the client.

While you are taking notes during the session, (since all minds are in constant communication) you are also receiving information or insights used to make recommendations, which lead them to make the necessary changes for then to achieve self-healing and a better quality of life.

Beyond just telling them to drink and apply orin, your clients count on you for answers to tough health challenges, guidance and relief from stress and concerns.

Practice. Practice. Practice. After the session ends, review your notes. Use this time to replay the session (in your mind) and find any corrections to be made in your teaching, listening, or coaching skills.

Be sure to acknowledge the good work that your client is doing. Acknowledgement for your good work will come later.

After learning these steps from guiding several clients through successful sessions, this will become second nature to you. The day will come when you will know confidently and with certainty that you give the most "perfect" advice and treatment suggestions for every client.

When working with clients, let them know that you will start the session or consultation with an orin toast or communion as a way to honor their water, their UT journey and allow Spirit to guide the session.

9.2.20 Session with a male client from India

Client: What orin application would you suggest I use to get started, Sir?

Sage: What health condition made you decide that orin therapy was right for you?

Client: My energy is low, difficulty with digestion and I get brain fog.

Sage: Lets make this simple. Go pee. Collect every drop in a container like a jar or cup. Take a sip and hold it in your mouth for a few minutes. Swish or gargle the golden water while it is in the mouth. When you are ready, swallow.

Will you do this?

Client: Yes, I will.

Sage: Try this a few times a day as a way to get used to the drinking protocol or application. As soon as you get comfortable with drinking orin orally, then comes nose drinking. In our next session, you will be taught this protocol. This is a direct route to the pituitary or master gland and all centers of the brain. With a brain that is free from calcification and hydrated sinuses, your thinking will become clear and sharp again.

Sage: Topical applications are simple and very effective. Why wait? While you are practicing drinking orin, try using the protocols for external application. Soak a washcloth or cotton ball in orin. For example: massage or dab orin with a cotton ball or washcloth into any affected skin areas, liver area, feet, scalp and any area that feels sore or needs improvement. Are you willing to try this? All of the UT protocols are my UT books. *

Client: Yes

Sage: Try an orin foot soak. Get a soft plastic 2-gallon tub (like a Tupperware brand). Fill tub with at least 2 quarts of orin that will cover the feet to the level of the ankles. Add hot water if you want the temperature of the orin to feel as comfortable as possible. Or just put in your feet and enjoy the cold stimulating effect until you the water is just right.

The more you can use full strength orin vs. diluted orin – the better. A diluted version still works well. It is just more of a subtle modality (homeopathic).

Have something to do while you are in the bathroom, like read a book, write in a journal or listen to music. You will be soaking for 30 minutes receiving the most benefits visualizing the medicine being delivered throughout the blood stream and cells. The entire foot soak protocol is explained in detail along with an instructional video in the book, Healing Water from Within* ©2018 and

Client: Sure Sir

Sage: When will you be starting?

Client: Today, Sir, for sure

Sage: Awesome. It will be at that time that your Journey   to Wellness begins.

Client: Yes, Sir. It will go right?

(Client sends screen shot of his face with red blotches across his cheeks.)

Client: I have it like this

Sage: You will learn to trust the water as well as your intuition. The healing will go quicker than you may imagine, my friend.

Client: How many times do I need to apply, Sir, before I start seeing any improvement? Teach me from your experience.

Sage: Drink orin every 3-4 hours. More often if condition is worse.

Client: Okay. How many days am I supposed

to do UT?

Sage: All the protocols are in both of my UT books. Making up a date for your healing to end is impossible to calculate.

Since the innate intelligence of the body is in control (and not you), *every healing happens its own timing.* It is not you or I who has that knowledge.

Meanwhile continue drinking orin, swishing or gargling and begin practicing topical protocols every day. Get back to me every 3-5 days. You'll be well and pleased very soon with your results. See if you can improve the quality of your diet as well as take time to relax often.

Remember: Orin Therapy is a lifetime practice that will prevent or cure an illness. Shivambhu is not a one time fix or remedy. It is not another "been there, done that" experience. How well we handle our emotions, raise the quality of our thoughts and how we manage our energy plays as much part in wellness as does practicing UT protocols.

9.2.20 session with
a female client from USA

Client: Hello, Brother I come to you seeking healing advice. The other day I used a Q-tip in my ear and now I cannot hear much. There is so much pain and it feels like half my head is underwater. There is much pressure. I was going to try garlic and urine. What are your thoughts?

Sage: First. Breathe. Good to hear from you, sister. Just use fresh or aged orin, skip the garlic (unless using garlic essential oil, which is optional). Do you know how to give yourself a urine ear rinse?

Client: Yes. I do not have aged at this time.

Sage: Not a problem. Use fresh orin that is collected during the day. Its best to use orin soaked Q-tips for ear cleaning only on the outer areas and never put it in the ear canal.

Got a dropper bottle with a dropper?

Client: Yes, I do.

Sage: Great. Squeeze a dropper full into an

ear. Hold the orin in the ear as long as you can before tilting the head to the opposite side and draining the ear. If any orin pours down the side of your face, rub it on your face or hair.

Client: Would it be harmful to collect urine during menstruation?

Sage: Pee and period blood do not exit the body from the same place—urine exits from the urethra (which has sphincters so it can be controlled) while period blood exits from the vagina, which does not have sphincters, so it cannot be controlled.

Any decision to use orin at this time is up to each person.

Sage: No, using orin at this time *will not be harmful*. Fill dropper bottle with orin. Tilt head to one side and drop a dropper full of the water into the affected ear. Massage entrance to ear to help orin soak deeper into ear. Hold orin in the ear for as long as it feels comfortable. Then tilt head back to drain ear.

Orin collected during menstruation works just fine. Orin is from yellow blood plasma and not from red blood cells. Its chemistry is beyond that of a biological purification period.

Understand? Shivambhu goes past our limited understanding about our natural abilities and what's possible with self-healing. We have to learn to stretch the mind to realize that orin is called our *perfect medicine* for a reason.

Orin transcends our concerns about a "sick" body, gender, age or race. One of my UT colleagues drinks the orin of some of his female clients who have cancer, diabetes, AIDS and MS to prove to them that Orin is the cure, not the cause.

You got this?

Client: Yes, thank you very much.

Sage: During any menstruation cycle remember to use an orin compress over the pubic bone areas near the uterus and ovaries. An orin foot soak will nourish the entire body using the reflexology points in the feet, especially those points that correspond to the reproductive organs, glands and pelvis area around both ankles.

Sage: I love you. Do this for you!!! Get back to me please with your results in the next 3-4 days.

Client: Thank you

Sage: AbsorbOrinlutely

Chapter 15
Presenting your UT service professionally

First, remind yourself that you got healthy and well because you drink orin. It is the water of life that saved your life and is keeping you vital, strong and active.

Still concerned about your partner or parents disapproving or judging you for drinking pee? Know that your radiant health, true happiness and mental freedom is contagious. Walk your talk. Teach by example. Let them see you being true to yourself & committed to your wellbeing. They will come around soon. Hang in there. You earned your body, mind and health back from every drop of Shivambhu that passed your lips. Now, go tell the world.

Would you like to become a UT teacher, therapist or an author? What is the role of a teacher or therapist? Would you like to become the next successful Orin Therapy teacher or best-selling author?

Differences between teaching and counseling are especially notable as related to the goal.

Teaching is about establishing a goal, then giving information and possibly advice about a course of action.

Ideally the teacher conducts a needs assessment and identifies a specific learning gap, or challenge, and establishes a clear learning goal that bridges the learning gap.

Counseling is goal-oriented, but in a different way. Neither the counselor nor the client has an exact agenda or agreed upon goal. In most cases, the "goal "of the conversation goes beyond just making suggesting on practicing AUT protocols, but the inclusion of health and wellness practices for mental, emotional, physical and spiritual wellbeing.

In other words, both client and counselor, during their initial consultation assess the client's needs, use inquiry to gather basic information from various areas of their life, and decide if you are good match or would make a good team to move forward working together.

Role of the client

A teacher leads the interaction. As an expert, they give information or recommend a course of action. The teacher helps the client to achieve a skill (mastering orin therapy protocols and practices) or avoid a particular action.

Instead of eating mucus forming, acidic, inflammatory or human made foods, you'll suggest that they eat living foods, fast, take enemas or practice meditation.

A counselor encourages a client to do most of the talking while the counselor listens, often taking notes during the consultation. These notes give clues, insights and an understanding of the depth of a client's cause of their health condition.

The counselor facilitates the sessions. They do not make a decision for the client, and most certainly, the counselor does not give advice but rather makes general suggestions.

Sometimes, the client changes their mind on the course of action, and a counselor's responsibility is to support and assist them through this process.

The roles are very different between teaching and counseling. A teacher's main job is to talk and *instruct* while a client listens. A counselor's main job is to listen, guide and *empower* the client.

In short, the difference between teaching and counseling are the words *direction* or *facilitation*. Teaching focuses on *directing* an action; counseling focuses on *facilitating* decisions or next actions.

Using inquiry methods (see chapter 10).

While coming to the closure or completion of each session, be sure to allow time for the client to express or communicate anything especially if they are unclear about what was discussed or what to expect next.

Ask the client if they wish to schedule another session and go deeper into the healing work with you? This leads to the follow-up.

When you are both certain about doing more sessions then reschedule them in the next 5-7 days.

Every session is different and reveals something to the client that they may have missed in the previous session.

Be sure to ask or referrals.

Shivambhu is an intuitive water or medicine

Once you choose this lifestyle (or it chooses you) and you absolutely know what UT is doing for you, you will never quit the practice or look for something "better."

After gaining enough experience practicing AUT and are sure that you are ready, students and clients will seek you out.

How well do you practice using your intuition? According to the Merriam-Webster dictionary: Intuition is an ability to understand something immediately, without the need for conscious reasoning. It is the **power or faculty of attaining direct knowledge or cognition without evident rational thought and inference**.

Do you feel confident with your intuitive abilities?

Intuition is a tool. It is only as good as the person who uses it.

Start today; right where you are, and practice being more mindful of using intuition. Mastering the use of intuition, along with mastering conscious breathing, is not only pivotal to your well-being and your clients, but also to everyone you know and will cross paths during your life.

Breathe.

Know that your intuition, instantly giving you quick and ready insight, is always at your service to guide & keep the session on course, assist in making good choices in giving advice, suggesting lifestyle changes and co-creating the best sessions with every client.

Remember you are an instrument, bridge or guide for your client to do his or her own work with your assistance and cooperation.

Your work is not to save, protect, improve or change anyone, especially clients.

The sooner a client can throw away their psychological or mental crutches, concerns, doubts and fears and take responsibility for their self-health care, the faster they will heal and grow.

They always heal themselves

Most clients come to you out of desperation, have given up hope and faith in the medical system and are looking to you and UT as their last chance to save their life, reclaim their health and have any quality of life.

You may at times when being approached

by new clients, feel like a first responder, answering to emergency calls, which can tend to scare you.

After facilitating more and more sessions, this becomes second nature to you. You got this? *You got this!*

Now would be a good time to set this book down, take several deep connected breaths. Get re-centered and calm. Go pee if you must. Perhaps start shaking the body, take a shower, dancing, do yoga, singing, yelling, chanting, skipping, running or walking.

These are powerful tools to use either during a session or anytime during the day when you feel stuck, anxious, concerned, confused, and uncreative or in "no movement."

Breathe. Exhale. Repeat.

Keep in mind that on this path, we give a lot of thanks to the **golden blood plasma water** for constantly cleaning, purifying and washing away impurities in body/mind while leaving us feeling fresh, clear, calm, balanced and sane.

Chapter 16
Presenting your UT service professionally to the media. Some proven promos that will bring greater interest in your work

Whether you read this manual, were mentored by one of the UT Master teachers or felt intuitively that you are ready to become a UT Teacher, the moment comes when you simply know that you are a UT teacher.

For the sake of this chapter, let's move forward in time when you have guided or facilitated enough sessions as an "amateur" UT teacher/therapist that you feel ready to become a professional and let everyone know.

Congratulations

Now would be the time to get prepared, create an online presence with a website, print business cards, blog, social media page and possibly a YouTube type of platform. Marketing and promoting your services takes time and requires being proactive and networking.

One of the best ways to get known and gain the respect of readers and possible interested clients is by writing and posting articles and producing videos with UT content that demonstrates your knowledge of the subject.

Writing UT articles reveals your knowledge on the subject and perhaps that you may need to do more research to sharpen your grasp of Orin Therapy. The more you can post content in the dozens of UT Facebook groups, *the more you will get known* and create a growing number of followers.

At one point in time, critical mass is reached and clients reach out and contact you. There is such a great need for UT teachers and therapists that you will have no problems manifesting clients and students.

It did just this for me. Within the first month after my book was released to 12 worldwide Amazon distribution regions and 8 radio interviews later, my UT career and mission with Shivambhu went viral.

Whether you announce or promote your UT service or not, be prepared for prospects or curiosity seekers seeking you and asking for help using orin to heal themselves.

Here are some proven promos that are currently being used and is bringing interest in Orin Therapy for self-healthcare.

1. Discover your own free natural immunity booster!

A healthy immune system is your best defense during a flu season or a "pandemic." It relies on the strength of antibodies, vitamin D, Zinc and vitamin C.

The body blends these nutrients with 1,000's of substances into ultra filtered blood plasma water as your perfect medicine, it is also known as orin.

This ancient yogic self healthcare practice, called Shivambhu Kalpa (Urine Therapy), supports a strong immune system, nourishes every system and function of the body, defends you against viral attack or compromise and restores health and well-being.

It feels great to know about a free natural "alternative" without waiting for a vaccine or medication.

Oral and topical use of AUT eliminates stress, supports immune system function and restores health for free.

2. The good news is that you have been carrying your perfect medicine and elixir of life with you since birth.
You do not have to rely on the medical system or health food industry to make you well.

Discover the world's ultimate free immunity booster!

Urine Therapy (UT)

3. What if the medical folks lied to us about urine being a waste product and got is wrong?
What if, in fact, *orin is a panacea or cure-all* and a unique custom made healing water just for us?

Orin may be the answer to our prayers and health concerns.

For any questions about Orin Therapy or possible collaboration, contact (insert your name and contact details here).

4. The Best Immune Booster is also Free!

In these troubled times, it is a great relief to know that we have in our possession both the prevention and remedy for any illness, virus or a compromised immune system.

Auto Urine Therapy (AUT) is an ancient Ayurvedic yoga practice using one's orin (a sterile, natural, anti-viral and anti-bacterial substance) to maintain and restore one's health.

This is amazing!

The medical industry lied to us with propaganda about the nature of our orin as a way to keep the truth from humanity.

If you read this far, pay attention! There are countless AUT enthusiasts and devotees who are extremely grateful that drinking their own water was just the perfect medicine they were seeking. It was an answer to their prayers.

Because of their devotion to their UT practice, they have learned that no matter what health challenges they may face, UT does restore their health every time.

With the UT message being aired on radio & internet talk shows, TV stations, magazines, newspapers, growing number of UT books and an incredible network of 100,000's of advocates on social media platforms, over 30 million pee drinkers have been discovered and are being united.

With very little assistance from any publications or media, the UT movement continues to grow, prosper and stay alive in 50 known countries.

It is with a grateful and humble heart, as the founder and director of Shivambhu, non profit organization, UT author, master teacher and outspoken voice for Shivambhu, that I am fully committed and determined to assist in the "declassification" and acceptance of UT worldwide.

Drink the living water that Matters and share this message with everyone.

Let's entertain our minds by thinking and visualizing that our clients and ourselves are already healed. We are just cleaning up our mess with our personal holy water. Bless yourself by honoring your temple with a touch or drink of orin for the body.

Be sure to love and nurture yourself with rest and play.

Chapter 17
To charge or not to charge for your services

Whether to charge or not to charge for your service is up for you to decide. Do you find value in your professional Urine Therapy service knowing that you will meet and exceed your client's concerns and needs?

Do you intend for your clients to relax and trust you? This takes as long as it takes for a meaningful relationship to be built. Each consultation requires your patience, calmness, sensitivity and tolerance for a client.

Ultimately it is up to you to set the direction of the session. As with any form of therapy, you are the facilitator of every session or meeting. You are not to presume any role as a "healer," savior or authority for them. You are guiding them to have realizations, a break through, Ah ha moments and in turn motivate themselves to make the changes that you have recommended.

Since they are relying on you to get results, most of the work is done. The answers to the concerns that they came to you to heal or resolve will be revealed it to you.

Your work is to teach them how to activate their innate knowing abilities. Since you read this far into the Manual, you probably know how to teach students *how to know what they need to know when they need to know it.*

Simply remind yourself first. Then remind a client that as long as you are telling yourself "I don't know this or I don't know that about this or that," you are blocking any understanding of what you want to know. Breathe.

Begin now to discipline the mind by using this powerful declaration statement:

"I choose to know_____." Write it by hand and complete the sentence with what you wish to know.

Breathe. Exhale. Breathe. Let go of every idea in the mind.

The knowingness comes.

Now move confidently though this new moment as one who knows. The satisfaction comes when the client is self-motivated. When they truly get excited or inspired by their "Why" (the results they are seeking from AUT and your work), their success is assured.

You just made a best friend for life!

It is the health giving and liberating benefits from *Shivambhu*, which are inspiring millions of devotees across earth to keep up this practice every day.

Determine the value or fee for your UT sessions either based on what similar professionals are charging or what you think clients will be willing to pay you.

Ultimately the value of any service is based on the value the client receives from working with you. A payment is a form or expression of appreciation.

Offering a sliding scale fee is perfect for clients with financial exceptions. By selling multiple session packages, a client will not only save money on each session, but most importantly they will be making a commitment to do the work with you on a regular basis.

Regular sessions give a client the chance to monitor their progress and to feel that you are on their wellness team. They are more likely to do these practices and follow treatment and lifestyle suggestions during the week or time between sessions.

By scheduling every prepaid session on your calendar and on theirs, they will stay committed and be more proactive in doing the work and succeeding.

Be open to negotiating with any client who has a money concern.

Giving away a number of sessions *for free* will give you an opportunity to practice generosity as well as find out if you are really motivated by money or for the joy of providing a service. You can also learn how well you know about the subject as well as your ability to coach and guide others.

Marketing is very basic. Get the word out about who you are and what you have to offer both online, offline and in person.

Working with the media and social media will require doing some research into which related subjects they have covered. Your chances of being interviewed or having an article accepted are better when the media that interests you has covered UT before. If presented properly and content is relative to modern times, your chances of having your article published or being interviewed will be much higher.

Hint: they like to have references included in an article.

Whether you are keeping your marketing efforts local, national or international is up to you and tends to go at your own pace.

Your success in doing promotions increases by associating with colleagues and other UT teachers. By constantly studying and keeping current with the Shivambhu movement and new discoveries, and building close friends in the water community will be to your advantage.

Chapter 18
What the experts say about AUT

Enjoy articles by contributing educators, therapists and researchers

by Maa Tejomayee Devi (Mataji)

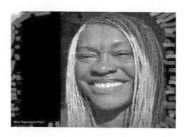

"Shivambu Kalpa (commonly known in modern times as "urine therapy") is an ancient holy science bestowed by the God Shiva to his consort, Goddess Parvati.

This ensemble of practices and

techniques were initially kept a secret only to be practiced by the seeker of truth, perfect health, divinity and ultimately physical immortality.

Since UT is often misunderstood by common human beings, Lord Shiva expressly recommended that it was "not for the ignorant," therefore keeping it secret.

Nevertheless, one can find its roots in most cultures and ancient traditions (holy scriptures), healing recipes and rituals as well. UT is indeed a wonderful thing and there is such perfection in human beings although UT is forgotten or unknown by the majority of the world.

UT is rejuvenating, healing and holds mystic powers for those who have the fortunate luck to discover it, fully explore UT and most of all, stay devoted to their daily UT practices for the long run.

UT is wisdom and a Tantra yogic sadhana or practice. You can find the numerous qualities it will bestow on the practitioner in the Shivambhu Kalpa (Damar Tantra)."

Divine Blessings Love and Light to all humanity
—Maa Tejomayee Devi (Mataji)*

Aged Urine by Harry Matadeen *

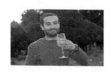

Your fresh orin, when contained and allowed to sit awhile, becomes what we call "aged." Like a fine wine, the medicinal powers of the fresh orin grows and grows the longer it is contained and allowed to sit. It is the most powerful medicine on earth.

What's going on?

Why does it grow in power and potency? What are the mechanisms I hear you cry. There are many, but the key ones which are alkaline, oxygen and high negative ions are explained in detail in Harry's books (Amazon).

In Harry's books and his unique style of writing, he answers questions like these about benefits and use of aged orin. (1) How do I age orin properly? (2) Does aged orin smell (3) Will sending loving thoughts to my orin make a difference? (4) Does aged orin get affected by diet? (5) Are there any other ways to increase the quality of my orin? (6) Do I need to drink fresh orin before doing aged orin? (7) What's that white stuff at the bottom of my aged orin?

Again, there's no such thing as *"bad" aged orin.* If it concerns you, you can scrape off any ugly looking things from the top that may appear, but I don't fear them, I drink and use everything.

Some of mine are so old now they get mushroom stuff on the top of them. At this point it's even more powerful than normal aged orin. I leave you with rich blessing and a big thank you.

I hope aged orin rewards you with optimal health and vitality, youthful vigor and a gratitude for life. We are blessed indeed with our own personal pharmacy and its power.

Thousands of years from now this knowledge of aged orin will be normal, it will be mainstream and used by everybody.

But until then, you my friend are a pioneer and I salute you. Thank you for carrying the torch forward and showing others the way. Those who use Orin Therapy and aged orin will always be standing on the right side of history.

God bless you.
—*Harry Matadeen*

Monica Schütt* on Aged Urine (see chapter 7 UT protocols)

Life is Water by George Johnson

Life is water.

We came to the world in water. When we were inside the womb of our mother, we drank the water. Where did it go?

We would pee it out and reabsorb it again. Why do you think babies are so gorgeous, happy, healthy, amazing soft skin? Because they have the best, most pure health of all people in the world.

The infinite creator is a genius providing us with such an amazing start in our life. The *powers that shouldn't be* think otherwise that we need to poison our children with vaccines and such.

Etymology explains the meaning of words from when it was created. Pharmacy is explained as maker of drugs, poison, spells. Does this sound like a company you would like to buy products from?

Once we remember and get back to life the way we started, reabsorbing our own fluids our life will transform.

Urine therapy is the most powerful healing therapy in the world. It is the fountain of youth. A guy told me that he had heard that Camel urine heals cancer, I told him right away urine from animals is being used in skin cream products, why do you think it makes the skin soft? Temporarily of course with these creams so you'll come back for more.

Urine is the elixir of life.

—George Johnson

Dr. David Jubb* on Urine Therapy

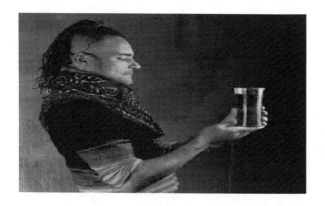

The most common complaint today is vascular dementia and poor micro circulation. Urea opens up blood vessels by shrinking water logged terrain. It is then that intestinal lesion is healed by B-vitamins made by friendly intestinal lifecolloid, of which the nitrogen from *urine therapy* is useful and such a practise shifts lifecolloid toward useful proto bacillus.

Arteriosclerosis is rampant in the modern world and nitreous oxide carbon dioxide are all smooth muscle dialators, of which Urine Therapy assists the intestine produce for you by assisting correct intestinal dysbiosis and accompanying layering of cholesterol inside artery walls. That's often one of the most important insights into Urine Therapy.

Seeing that all are born in amniotic fluid as I was growing up in the wilderness of Tasmania, I used urine to wash, clean and make dye for cloth. Kept listening to how the originals used urine therapy. Since the late seventies saw how urea is central to all molecular conditioning of cells including good skin creams.

I get the US therapeutic grade urea to put into a product made from jack beans.

Noticed that many cultures all were using Urine Therapy. The kidneys are a regulating essential element and not an organ of detoxification.

Once you start drinking or splashing urine on the skin and/or snorting this water through the nose, you should never stop. I've kept up a daily practice ever since. Urine purifies the blood. Urine Therapy assists in restoring vital cell salts.

Start by splashing or wetting skin with urine. Try gargling then snorting and drinking by starting with smaller amounts at first.

Best to include life giving enzymes in the diet and practicing calorie restriction. *Only eat one meal a day.*

Urine is the only thing you'd ever drink except for the moment after our birth, colostrum and breast milk. When growing up as an infant nothing is better than the nutrient benefits of Urine Therapy. Urine allows elements of the blood to get to the furthest regions of the human body. Blood ordinarily can't reach inside the nose and in the intestinal tract.

I've seen urine used as a subcutaneous lymphatic delivery. UT can stop the effects of a heart attack and turn an asthmatic or an allergic attack around. This provides antibodies and anti-toxin abilities to the body.

Urine senses overall conditions more than just a local condition as an immune force for an entire systemic effort to take care of you.

Luv, Dr Jubb xxx

Aged Urine by Dave Murphy*

Aged urine is that which has been stored for 8 days or more. When stored correctly, Urine can be kept indefinitely, and the older it gets the more effective it becomes.

To age urine, store fresh urine in a glass container with a gas permeable covering so that it can "breathe", for example, if using a bottle, then stop with a wad of cotton wool, if using a jar then cover with a piece of cloth held in place with an elastic band. Store in a cool place where it will not be disturbed

Urine is a "living" liquid, *it remains alive as long as you do*, and the stem cells (undifferentiated cells that can become anything within the body) that it contains, continue to divide and multiply while in storage. This makes "aged urine" a very powerful agent for healing cuts, burns, rashes, and inflammation or for any other topical use.

> **"Fresh urine is perfect for long term daily use as it boosts bodily performance"**
> **—Fabian Farquharson**

Why do I drink my own urine? By Leah Sampson, Standing White Buffalo*

I was just asked, why do I drink my own urine? Here was my response: "At the age of 12, in 1984, I was diagnosed with chronic migraines. In 1988, asthma. 1998, hypothyroidism, and tendinitis in both shoulders, right elbow and right wrist. In 2009, I was morbidly obese at 250 pounds and while pregnant, diagnosed with cervical cancer. In 2012, fibromyalgia and kyphoscoliosis with mild degenerative disc disease, bilateral carpal tunnel and ulnar nerve entrapment. In 2013, Complex Post Traumatic Stress Disorder. In 2016, 15% of my body sustained first and second-degree steam burns.

I drink my urine daily, excluding when menstruating, because urophagia is an ancient indigenous practice that heals and is a procedure that in 2012 my family doctor agreed I could do because nothing else we were doing to combat my complex medical conditions, including using six different daily prescriptions, was working.

I drink my urine because I am a registered North American treaty status Indian with Muscowpetung Saulteaux First Nation, and it is part of my culture. One of my grandfathers, Dakota Santee Sioux Chief Inkpaduta survived battles at Wounded Knee, as well as the Battle of Little Bighorn (Custer's Last Stand). He also survived small pox. I'm willing to deduce that my grandfather drank or used his own urine topically in order to do that.

I drink my own urine because I read Martha Christy's book entitled Your Own Perfect Medicine and noted the medical studies that confirmed it worked.

Urine is my body's own perfect medicine, or amniotic fluid for me complete with stem cells that helps maintain my health, weight, cognitive function, reduce inflammation & allergies, prevents cancer regrowth and after receiving first and second degree steam burns in 2016. It helps me regrow skin, without scars, as well as heal wounds substantially faster. It's also helping me improve my eyesight.

Medical doctors have informed me that they can not tell that I was ever morbidly obese, or have the diseases and chronic illnesses that I have been diagnosed with. Urophagia is one of the many reasons why.

I drink my own urine since discovering that babies are born with soft skin. Fetuses drink their own urine while in their mothers womb. Within nine months, babies have evolved from a sperm and an egg, to a fish, known as a foetus that drinks its own urine and then they evolve into an air breathing being that is able to walk and speak within a year. That's a miracle, and urine, also known as amniotic fluid, is part of that miracle.

Society pays money to drink acidic chemical fluids from beverage companies and they don't know the source of these ingredients. I know what goes into my body and that my urine is free. Why wouldn't I drink a fluid that I know who made it, where it comes from, and that it also produces miracles? *It seems nonsensical to me to not drink my own urine.*

I drink my own urine because I choose to live and evolve. Dr. Masaru Emoto proved scientifically that water has memory, urine is distilled water with memory that has been filtered by the body.

Drinking, washing and using my urine daily is also a very sustainable eco-friendly water conservation practice. Water is life. The water on our planet is only becoming more polluted and is more expensive than gasoline. What's the cost of water going to be in 20 years? My water is becoming cleaner and cleaner every day.

I drink my urine because I became sick and tired of being sick, fat, tired and nearly dead. I was staring death in the face and I decided I wanted to live, those are the reasons why I drink my urine, and I don't care who knows, because it works, at least, it's working for me.

My multi-disciplinary medical team has advised me that I should not have survived what I have survived and that my recovery is remarkable. I'm an indigenous woman that has survived generations of wars, and severe domestic violence that has not been murdered or gone missing. Doctors keep telling me that I should've been dead and that there's no medical reason or explanation why I am alive.

I recently had a professor of neurology inform me that my cognitive function was remarkable and that which he had never seen before. I can only attribute my success and survival in part to practising urophagia.

There's more reasons, however; that's why I drink my own urine

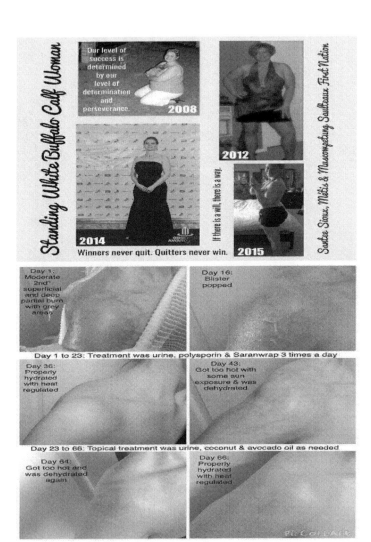

Standing White Buffalo Calf Woman

Saulteaux Sioux, Métis & Muscowpetung Saulteaux First Nation

Our level of success is determined by our level of determination and perseverance. **2008**

If there is a will, there is a way.

2012

2014

Winners never quit. Quitters never win. **2015**

Day 1: Moderate 2nd° superficial and deep partial burn with grey areas

Day 16: Blister popped

Day 1 to 23: Treatment was urine, polysporin & Saranwrap 3 times a day

Day 36: Properly hydrated with heat regulated

Day 43: Got too hot with some sun exposure & was dehydrated

Day 23 to 66: Topical treatment was urine, coconut & avocado oil as needed

Day 64: Got too hot and was dehydrated again

Day 66: Properly hydrated with heat regulated

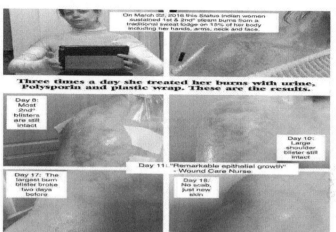

On March 22, 2016 this Status Indian women sustained 1st & 2nd° steam burns from a traditional sweat lodge on 15% of her body including her hands, arms, neck and face.

Three times a day she treated her burns with urine, Polysporin and plastic wrap. These are the results.

Day 8: Most 2nd° blisters are still intact

Day 10: Large shoulder blister still intact

Day 11: "Remarkable epithelial growth" - Wound Care Nurse

Day 17: The largest burn blister broke two days before

Day 18: No scab, just new skin

If you don't believe in miracles perhaps you forgot that you are one that drank its own urine for nine months before being born.

Urine Therapy by Alquivar Marin*

What is urine?

There are approximately 170 liters of blood are filtered in the kidneys per day, but only approximately 1.4 liters are excreted. More than 90% of the water is reabsorbed. Each kidney weighs approximately 141 grams and is made up of more than 1,200,000 nephrons or filters, that is, more or less 2,400,000 filters or nephrons.

If we spread the nephrons one after the other, it would measure about 80 kilometers. The first part of the nephron separates part of the plasma from the blood that is forced through delicate capillaries, when these expand with the heartbeat, red cells, white cells, protein units and vitamin units and other relatively small particles.

In the second process or stage of filtration of the nephron, it again absorbs more than 90% of plasma, leaving behind what we know as urine. It was found in 1992 at the Hayashibara Institute of Biochemistry in Japan, that urine is a blood product, not a waste of useless substance.

In reality urine is the most miraculous and mysterious juice in the world that your body made for your body, to be used as medicine and at the same time as natural nutrition.

Urine is a sterile fluid while it is in the urethra. Urine has more than two thousand (2,000) organic compounds and many of them are specific for each body. Its main ingredient is water (60-98%) urine contains hormones that go from the pineal gland to the sex glands, it also contains steroids, proteins, minerals, vitamins, enzymes, antioxidants, antibodies, antitoxins, muscle cells, muscle tissues, cellular tissues, endotoxins and exotoxins that are produced by the viruses, bacteria and microbes that live in our body.

For all this, it is much better to drink any or all of our urine and not consume it with anything artificially or chemically made by man. It is made by the most sophisticated laboratory made by God herself and not by man like the laboratory called the human body.

To all brave women and men who practice Urine Therapy, I bow to you.

The cure lives within us
by Cayce Kaban*

What are your ailments?

Are you seeking a cure?

Are you given treatments

That leave you unsure?

Most remedies relieve us

But that doesn't matter

Masking the symptoms

When the cure's in our bladder

The poisons consumed

Are always there

It's in our food

Water and air

Some we control

No need to assume

It's simply based

On what we consume

If you don't feel good

Do you know why?

Do you pop a pill?

And hope you don't die?

The cure lives within us

Just look and see

It's very simple

Start drinking your pee

Chapter 19
Shivambhu Master Teachers and superstars

Here is the most up to date roll call

Dr. Tal Schaller, UT teacher (France) 45 years

Dr. Rakshak Mal Lodha, UT teacher/advisor (India) 50+ years

Dr. Raojiibhai Manibhai Patel, Manav Mootra (AUT) 1963

Dr. G.K. Thakkar, Shivambhu Gita 1996

S.S. Saraswati, Amaroli

Trustees of Water of Life Foundation (based in India & worldwide)

C.P. Mithal Miracles of Urine Therapy

Coen van der Kroon, (Holland) The Golden Fountain; The Complete Guide to Urine Therapy 1993

Brother Sage, (Texas) Healing Water from Within 2018, Manual for Urine Therapy Teachers 2020

Leonard Orr, (Virginia) The Secrets of Youthing 1994

Andrew Norton Webber

Dr. Bunmi Sumoila

George Johnson

Dr. David Jubb, (Tasmania) author and lecturer on UT

Harold W. Tietze, Urine, The Holy Water

Martha Christy, Your Own Perfect Medicine 1999

J.W. Armstrong, (England) The Water of Life 1944

Beatrice Barnett, Urine Therapy: It May Save

Your Life

Flora Peschek-Bohmer, PHD, Urine Therapy, Nature's Elixir for Good Health 1997

Doc Mike Witort, (Chicago) UT teacher 22 years

Martin Lara, Uropathy 1999

Harry Matadeen, (UK) Aged Urine Discovery of the Century 2019

Lee Robert Moulson

Monica SchÜtt, author of many UT articles

Dainis W. Michel, urine-therapy.org

Alquivar Marin, www.orinoterapia.org

Dr. Roselyn Hanson

Cayce Kaban

Allegedly Dave Murphy, www.allegedlydave. com

Troy Casey, Certified Healthnut, Youtube. com/user/certifiedhealthnut

Steven Williams (Urine Aid documentary), www.urineaid.com

URINE AID IS A RARE LOOK INTO THE CONTROVERSIAL WORLD OF URINE THERAPY. WITH DOCUMENTATION DATING BACK 3000BC TO THE ANCIENT EGYPTIAN EBER'S PAPYRUS.
URINE THERAPY IS ONE OF THE OLDEST FORMS OF HEALTH CARE. BOTH FASCINATING AND TABOO, THIS DOCUMENTARY EXPLORES THE CONFRONTING SUBJECT OF DRINKING URINE FOR MEDICINAL PURPOSES.

Anthony AK King (musician, director of Water of Life Symposium), www.youtube.com/channel/UCwPCpLNwnCOjFLo9m3fuooQ

Sandy Rodgers

Fabian Farquharson

Stampana Osenotse

Leah Sampson

Shirley of Shirley's Wellness Café, shirleys-wellness-cafe.com/UT/Urine

Ruby D. Karyo

Dr. Phillips, Omad Orin Looper

John DePass (Toronto, Canada), HiEndFitness Coach

Bryan Justice

Chapter 20
The Future of the Shivambhu movement and Urine Therapy

There is an increasing worldwide interest in becoming an Orin Therapy teacher. This is resulting in the creation of UT schools, educational programs, home study classes and conferences.

Our voices are being heard.

The Shivambhu movement is growing. There is still so much more work to do as our message is being spread mostly through social media, radio, TV shows and interviews.

Everyday more are taking this message and mission "to the streets and to the people who need a miracle." This has a been an organically growning "grassroots" movement up until 2020.

Moved by the healing of their own bodies, courageous individuals like you are putting aside concerns and fears and offering a life saving remedy by telling their friends and loved ones about their discovery of AUT.

Are you among these Shivambhu warriors?

As billions of people desperately seeking answers to their serious illness and wellbeing become more disappointed by the medical establishment, it will be up to us to speak up and take action. We need to continue sharing the Shivambhu message to all of humanity.

Let this be the day that world governments and their media tell the people of the world the truth about AUT.

Through spreading the education and awareness of AUT, the Shivambhu organization will be producing several AUT educational and instructional projects for 2021-2022 to empower everyone in this life changing practice.

Outreach programs, local water community meetings, support groups and UT teaching and therapy centers are being established in Africa, USA, UK, Germany, Australia and other countries.

Shivambhu's documentaries, trainings and research findings will be taught in schools, universities, churches, AA meetings, recovery centers, senior centers, wellness centers, websites and movie theaters across the world. Our tools are making AUT topics engaging for young and old viewers which is sparking excitement for further study.

With the training and confidence gained by upcoming UT teachers and therapists, many more are able to help their clients in their recovery to restore their health and achieve a better quality of life.

We continue to be blessed with countless numbers of Shivambhu enthusiasts joining us with their time, talent, energy and voices to the movement of all movements. Your devotion to UT practices and compassion for sisters and brothers is greatly appreciated and needed now more than anytime in history. The wisdom and ability for all humanity to take self healing into their own hands is changing the health care system on this planet forever.

Shivambhu is here to bring health freedom to many generations living today and well into the future.

Those with questions on how to join Shivambhu in its worldwide mission or have any suggestions, donations, proposals or ideas to further our work, you can reach us through Shivambhu.org.

"Following the Shivambhu Trail documentary" will travel the world with Brother Sage, assistant and a camera crew spreading the Shivambhu message along with orin therapy stories and recording inspiring news from people on the streets across the world.

Spin-offs will come after this book is published, which will include radio; television and Internet talk show interviews and articles. More respected celebrities will be coming forward and lending their names and reputations by endorsing AUT for the world to discover this practice for themselves.

Shivambhu will be producing Live-streaming webinars teaching UT courses from beginners UT 101 classes though master teacher level. They will also be offering Zoom UT conference calls with a Q & A format for audience participation.

We will be filming Brother Sage and the Shivambhu team hosting tables at popular public gathering places and events. Enjoy watching us presenting and dialoging with individuals as we introduce AUT and answer all questions about it.

There is a growing interest in becoming an Orin Therapy teacher in the United States and across the planet. This will result in the creation of Orin Therapy schools, educational programs, and "un-certification."

The term "un-certification" describes orin therapy practitioners who are prequalified from years of direct personal experience and results backed by their Shivambhu Lifestyle and remarkable health. These are all the credentials you will ever need. UT teachers will be grandfathered in by their commitment to share this important work. A percentage of the proceeds from fundraisers for the Shivambhu organization will go to causes and individuals who make a difference in the world. The purchase of property, housing, and Shivambhu headquarters will be established as The Purification and Retreat Center of the Pacific.

The Future of Auto Urine Therapy

The power of AUT gets confirmed by a "medically" controlled, double blind study. These lab test results will become the Gold standard for AUT's acknowledgement as the perfect medicine for humanity. Many peer reviewed published articles begin appearing on Universities and Medical websites and in Natural Healing publications.

Shivambhu, nonprofit organization, will be blessed with a wealthy philanthropist who not only sponsors the double blind study, they finance all of the staff, directors and projects for Shivambhu. This financial source has no economic or political interest in orin being tested.

They will not be motivated by profit from orin products, which ironically can't be patented or owned.

Since orin is the least controllable substance on earth, it is impossible to derive any monetary profit from it; therefore, our angel philanthropist, invested $100,000's to do the study.

The double blind study confirmed that laboratory tests are unnecessary in order to determine which virus is causing an infection and Orin Therapy is beneficial for human health.

As word spreads about AUT, many laboratory owners and technicians will be out of work.

Consequently, the pharmaceutical companies that make antibiotics as well as pharmacies and stores that sell antibiotics(including health food stores selling natural plant sources of antibiotics) are cutting back on their workforce and may possibly close their businesses because there is no need to use antibiotics anymore.

Prime Minister Narendra Modi of India declares Urine Therapy, as an acceptable form of self-healthcare, to the entire nation of India.

Governments will include UT in the curriculum in all the medical and educational institutions. Hospitals and healthcare providers will provide AUT as their number one treatment. All states and countries will give official recognition to AUT.

There will be a cooperation and coordination between different healthcare disciplines to assist in overcoming all illnesses and contributing to the happiness, well-being and health of humanity.

We will become self reliant as people find out about this basic and natural therapeutic practice, which is safe, sure, simple and free. This is the gift of life, known as Shivambhu or Orin Therapy.

Photo of people in the future holding communion in public places

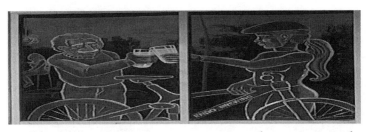

Recent reply to a water brother in South Africa @ UT training, UT centers in Africa and "certification."

You can get my previous book, Healing Water from Within (tinyurl.com/OrinTherapy) or as a digital color copy direct from me. There are currently no formal training centers in S. Africa. There are a growing number of UT practitioners scattered across Africa. The strong water families in Botswana, Nigeria and Kenya are working on a UT conference with me as a guest speaker.

However, as I have written this manual, you become self-certified after mastering UT protocols and have experience mentoring and teaching others.

With AUT, it doesn't matter the name of a disease or story about it, lab tests or personal beliefs, Shivambhu brings healing, miracles and answers to prayers.

Chapter 21
Humor as a therapeutic adjunct to AUT does make a difference

Smiling not only increases one's face value, smiling produces endorphins and happy molecules. While dealing with the "controversial" subject of drinking one's pee and sharing AUT with sick people you wish to help, it will take a sense of humor as well as a sensitivity to earn the acceptance by "prospects and newbies on the UT path."

The *Pisscabulary of Orinisms was included in the book, Healing Water from Within (Tinyurl.com/OrinTherapy) along with piss cartoons, pee jokes, celebrities discussing drinking pee or people singing pee drinking songs was for readers to learn how to lighten up when presenting UT to anyone.

Humor and piss puns produce a temporary shift in the mind in its attempt to take in a new idea, particularly one that challenges our perception of reality or beliefs learned from "trusted" sources.

While a person is going through mental gymnastics to be able to understand and integrate this new idea (known as the "sorting out" period), AUT, as an idea is worth considering.

This must sink deeper into the mind until they "get it."

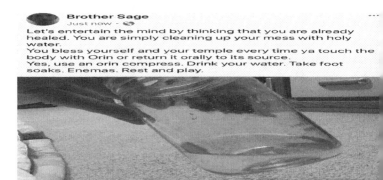

Brother Sage
Just now ·

Let's entertain the mind by thinking that you are already healed. You are simply cleaning up your mess with holy water.
You bless yourself and your temple every time ya touch the body with Orin or return it orally to its source.
Yes, use an orin compress. Drink your water. Take foot soaks. Enemas. Rest and play.

Humor is the key that opens the mind. It spices and lightens up any apparent difficulties. Humor, like a powerful laser light, penetrates even the most guarded of minds, allowing news ideas to be planted in a now fertile soil.

One pioneer in laughter research claimed

it took ten minutes on a rowing machine for his heart rate to reach the level it would *after just one minute of hearty laughter*.

Ten minutes of laughter can easily produce two hours of pain-free sleep as well as a mind that is free from worry.

It has been shown in several studies that the ability to laugh raises the level of infection-fighting antibodies by the body as well as boosts the level of immune cells. Your body responds incredibly well to the effects of belly laughs.

Orin, especially during looping (either sip looping or all out looping), increases antibodies, nourishes the nervous system (especially the adrenal glands), normalizes work of blood vessels and lowers blood pressure.

Adding comedy, humor and laughter reactivates, amplifies and enhances the body's strength as it brings positive effects.

Regardless of whether laughter actually does improve your health or boosts your energy, it undeniably improves your quality of life. Enjoying laughing is the reason to laugh.

Being pissed on is more therapeutic then staying pissed off

Get hip by learning an hilarious NEW Orin language. It ispacked with piss-rich puns and new Orin words with definitions. Learn it today, it won't be conPisscated and you will not be pissing away your time.

Breathe. Exhale and release all pressure from your belly, mind, bladder and intestines.

Here's a pissTacular idea that will pissillitate your Co-orin-ation with others. Pee puns are guaranteed to take you beyond the known Orin-a-Verse, the OrinOsphere where Shivambu devotees gather.

The worldwide water family openly and sincerely show their PissPect and love for each other.

In my experience, I feel everyone's love and gratitude for hearing this message in the most PeeFect way. Just Pee HappPee, Pee Active and drink yourPee today.

Today's Mantra: I now Pee easily, effortlessly and on time.

I release, relax and am present when I pee.

Are we having a MagPissadent time now?

Urine good hands with your own water, just trust and flow with it.

Hey, if they can't take a joke....you know what to do.

Have you come aboard the Orin Wave before it becomes the Big Change? Come on in, the water is fine.

Either get pissy drinking orin or get busy sinking.

HemPeeNomics—What happens with a hemp farmer uses Orin in his filed. His plants and income peecome PeeNormous.

Was it Mary Poppins who sang a verse that contained the word, exPeeAladoshas?

Simply let the PissCabulary of Orin-isms(* resources) fill up your joy tank and you will never be Piss poor again.

Chapter 22
Shivambhu a 501C3 non-profit organization Shivambhu Hut, the First alternative Social Media platform focused just on UT

Shivambhu's mission is to support and educate individuals in taking responsibility for their personal well-being through the daily practice of auto-urine therapy.

To tip the tipping point, the increasing cosmic energy or light wave is here. It is visible as a golden liquid structure known as Shivambhu. To reach as many minds as possible, messengers are using their voices & platforms, like Social Media, TV, radio and books.

Our efforts to bring the Shivambhu message to local residents is paying off.

When channel 9News aired a story in 2019 at one of our Urine Therapy meetup of Colorado meetings at the main Boulder Library, it released an avalanche of attention, discussion & growing interest in Orin Therapy. There has not only been over 23,000 views of this story since this TV story aired, but this also spun off to dozens of interviews and stories about UT showing up across the planet.

Looks like the Urine Therapy of Colorado meetup group keeps spreading. Our recent meeting drew the attention of a 7News journalist. After airing the story, several affiliate news stations, ESPN sports & Newsweek presented their version of the story.

Within a week, Brother Sage was contacted and interviewed on a health show based in China Sama 0ne on One with John*

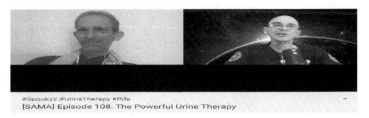

#Spooky2 #UrineTherapy #Rife
[SAMA] Episode 108: The Powerful Urine Therapy

All responses, positive or negative continue

bringing more energy to this sacred mission & message.

Shivambhu organization has positioned itself as a major education and awareness leader or branch in the Shivambhu movement.

Some of the work of Shivambhu is to bring the education and awareness to local communities. By taking the Shivambhu message and mission offline, many more who do not use the internet can be reached.

Working with local UT enthusiasts and the local media stations creates a stronger local presence for the city and state. With regular UT meetings, new people can learn about UT while being in a room with devoted UT people and gain by their experiences and wisdom.

These local UT communities will learn how to introduce UT to newbies, become UT teachers and promote their groups (the gift of the water of life) in person, online and with the local media.

Having a local support group brings enthusiasm for Shivambhu by creating a safe space for folks to open up about their UT journey, successes, failures and new ideas on making UT presentations. Every water sister and water brother who meets with others forms an unbroken friendship for life.

Will you take a stand with Shivambhu and the Shivambhu movement?

Invite your friends to join us at our own alternative social media platform known as the Shivambhu Hut. Here you can ask questions, dialogue with fellow UT practitioners and post UT content for members to enjoy. Here at the "Hut" you can read articles and watch educational and entertaining UT videos.

All Hut members, which we affectionately refer to as "water family," are encouraged to contribute any content relating to UT topics that are found on the site. Use your writing skills and passion for this precious water, to educate others which furthers the awareness and message of AUT across earth.

Supporting Shivambhu financially, energetically or through collaborating helps with logistics, promotions, productions, public outreach and day to day work in building, maintaining & growing a global humanitarian mission.

Bless you for coming home to our water family and especially coming home to you.

Let us know today

Much water love
Brother Sage

References

Ch. 4   Melatonin from early morning urine drinkingpubmed.ncbi.nlm.nih.gov / 1787809 /

Ch. 6 pH range of urine from Wikipedia en.wikipedia.org / wiki / urine

Ch. 8   Research and Clinical Studies

Urine Therapy briefing for Scientists 2012 https:/ / pdfs.semanticscholar.org / d091 / c3c5e14af730c31fbbf3dd7fdb4061f6f187.pdf

Excerpt from 2001 Article by Biomedx with passages from

Your Own Perfect Medicine by Martha Christy

100 Golden Facts about urine

www.factretriever.com / urine-facts

Testimonials

UT testimonials for hands, feet and nails

peoplespharmacy.com/articles/urine-therapy-for-hands-feet-nails

Testimonials from Shirley's Wellness Cafe

shirleys-wellness-cafe.com/UT/Urine

Testimonials from clients of Jagdish R. Bhurani
urinetherapy.in/customer_testimonials.aspx

Testimonials from UrineCure.orgurinecure.org/testimonials

Albert Woolridge UT testimonial

drive.google.com/file/d/1X9leCKp3lBpxu9z-mY4xRjJSjeE9uI1Xy/view

The Practical Uses of Pee

Resources

Social Media groups

Shivambhu Hut https://shivambhu.org/shivambhu-hut

Facebook Groups

Urine Therapy: The Real Universal Remedy

Urine Therapy Is New World Water

Shivambu: (Facebook)

Urine Therapy No Trolls Edition (Facebook)

The Activation of the Philosopher's Stone Aged Urine Therapy

(Facebook)

Urinoterapia Urinoterapia

Teachers

Moraji Desai, former Prime Minister of India

Dr. Rakshak Mal Lodha (Facebook)

Andrew Norton Webber on Urine Therapy (Youtube)

Dr. Roslynn Hansen (Facebook)

Brother Sage BrotherSage.com

Manjushree Abhinav (Facebook)

Dr. David Jubb   en.wikipedia.org/wiki/David_Jubb

Allegedly Dave Murphy   Allegedly Dave

Leah Sampson Facebook.com/standing-whitebuffalo/ Twitter.com/standingwhitebu Instagram.com/standingwhitebuffalo Muscowpetung.com Youtube.com/watch?v=t_8Zq_ZejZ0&feature=youtu.be

Dainis W. Michel urine-therapy.org

Troy Casey www.TroyCasey.com

Kelly Ra Saliba (Youtube)

Samuel G. Cohen Drinkingthroughthenose.com

Doc Mike Witort www.wakeupwell.org (630-613-8537) wakeupwell1@gmail.com

Dr. Vijay & Prof. Indira Gupta cires.colorado.edu/fellow-emeritus-past-fellow/vijay-gupta

Media Coverage

Denver Channel 9 story aired June 12, 2019

https://www.9news.com/article/news/local/group-in-boulder-drinks-their-own-pee-for-health-benefits/73-80277854-becf-4e0e-bade-9b2e2745ed1e

Denver Channel 7 story aired Jul 23, 2019

Thedenverchannel.com/news/national/a-urine-therapy-group-in-colorado-touts-the-benefits-of-drinking-your-own-pee-doctors-disagree

Organizations

Shivambhu hivambhu.org

Shivambhu Hut shivambhu.org/shivambhu-hut

Urine Good Humor at the Shivambhu Hut Shivambhu-hut.mn.co/topics/1640719

Authors

Water of Life by J.W. Armstrong

Manav Mootra by Raojibhai Manibhai Patel

Auto-Urine Therapy by Jagdish R. Bhurani

Wonders of Urotherapy;Urine Therapy as a Universal Cure by Dr. G.K. Thakkar

Amaroli by Dr. Tal Schaller

Alquivar Marin El Jugo Milagroso www.orinoterapia.org

The Miracles of Urine Therapy by Beatrice Barnett

Your Own Perfect Medicine by Martha Christy

Urotherapy by Martin J. Lara

Aged Urine by Harry Matadeen

Drinking Urine Through the Nose by Samuel G Cohen www.drinkingthroughthenose.com

Golden Fountain: The Complete Book on

Urine Therapy by Coen van der Kroon

Healing Water from Within ©2018 Brother Sage Tinyurl.com/OrinTherapy

PissCabulary of Orin-isms can be found in *Healing Water fom Within*

Videos - Instructional and Entertaining

Diffusing with Orin demo:

www.facebook.com/brothersage/videos/10156658669776529/?extid=3MX6zKKn-BYsqaw9F&d=n

Ear, eye, nose & multiple protocols youtube.com/watch?v=67_Pa585SRQ

Ch. 11 UT shortcut teaching method www.facebook.com/brothersage/videos/10157125188186529

Tongue cleaning demo www.facebook.com/brothersage/videos/10157102159071529/

Events

Water of Life Symposium 2021 Las Vegas, NV wateroflifesymposium.com

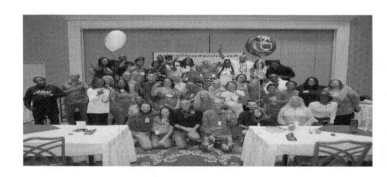

Return to Purity 2020
Baja California, Mexico

Urine Therapy Conference 2020
Botswana, Africa

Last word from Author

Since the first release of Urine Therapy books in 1944, rather than the doubt and criticism one would expect to encounter, there was tens of thousands of people who willingly accepted the information in these books.

Thanks to somebody having the love, courage and wisdom to take the time to share UT with others, there are currently over 30 *known* million Shivambhu enthusiasts worldwide.

Many people (including doctors) are coming forward to talk about their own UT experiences or about news stories they've read that talk about using urine medicinally, orally and topically and in survival situations. After reading over these reports, and looking at all of the other many studies on urine therapy, I couldn't help thinking, "Why didn't anyone ever tell us?" Keep the Shivambhu faith, dear ones. Keep doing an awesome job at spreading the message.

Glad we have been blessed with our water family.

About the Author

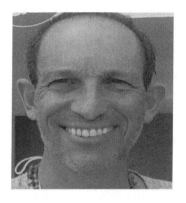

Brother Sage has been passionate about writing and producing books, *Conversations That Matter* talk show, articles, artwork, murals and videos that inspire, bring insights and transform people his whole life.

As well as being a prolific writer, he continues a successful wellness practice in Boulder, Colorado, which began in 1979. Brother Sage is an international wellness consultant, popular guest on dozens of radio / TV shows and facilitator/producer of purification retreats and community gatherings.

Brother Sage's Urine Therapy accolades

PhD in Urine Therapy 2018 granted by Vijay Gupta,* Professor Emeritus of Hydrology: Water Sciences at University of Colorado, Boulder, Colorado.

International Liaison for Water of Life Symposium 2018 appointed by Anthony A.K. King*

Produced local Urine Therapy of Colorado Meet-up groups held at the main library in Boulder, Colorado

Founder/Director of Communications for Shivambhu, 501c3, non profit organization 2019*

Interviewed elder UT Teachers, Dr. Rakshak Mal Lodha, Dr. Tal Schaller, Dr. David Jubb and Doc Mike Witort.

Conversations with UT superstars, Ruby Karyo, Leah Sampson, Harry Matadeen, Samuel G. Cohen and Kelly Ra, Henry Draper, Fabian Farquharson, John DePass, Tugce Zaloglu, Weedu Shivambu, Dr. Bunmi Sumoila, Stampana Osenotse, Manjushree Abhnav, Dr. Roslynn Hansen, Anthony AK King, Dr. Beauty Mwera Muzadzi and Maa Tejomayee Devi

Endorsements

Brother Sage is dedicated to Urine Therapy and serving all human beings in becoming healthy and well. He did lot of research on Urine Therapy.

I recommend this book written by Brother Sage for all medical colleges to teach the subject of Urine Therapy to medical students so people of the whole world shall be healthy forever. Urine Therapy is very effective in preventing and treating most diseases and has no side effects at all.

Urine is our best health insurance. UT gives us a sanitizer, auto vaccine and much more.

Urine is the nectar of life.
I have had experience in urine therapy for more than 50 years, creating countless followers all over world."
Regards

Dr Rakshak Mal Lodha

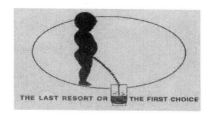

THE LAST RESORT OR THE FIRST CHOICE

"Brother Sage has accurately assembled key information of this ancient science of self-care and self-health practiced worldwide. The manual offers a roadmap covering education, research, service and outreach aspects to benefit all advocates. All educational institutions need to carry this timely message forward to help the global humanity."Professor Emeritus Vijay Gupta   The University of Colorado Boulder, CO., 80309

"Zindabad" "Long Live Shivambhu!"
Indira Bhatt Gupta

In India, urine therapy is called "Shivambhu."

Thanks to our Shivambhu rishi (Brother Sage), great devotee, propagator and mighty supporter of the <u>Shivambhu movement</u>* through his non profit organization, Shivambhu and centenarian former Prime Minister of India, respected (late) Morarji Desai (who boldly and emphatically declared before the world that he drank his own urine regularly, and that was the secret of his longevity and exuberant health) that this most valuable and beneficial information is being given to you today through this book.

Manual for Urine Therapy Teachers & Therapists©2020 will prove to be a boon to poor countries. Shivambhu is capable of curing a host of diseases ranging from a common cold to cancer, arthritis and diabetes to AIDS. Otherwise, UT would have remained hidden in some unknown quarters and the entire mankind would have been deprived of Shivambhu.

Really speaking, late Shri Morarjlbhai by his frank and honest declaration has accorded world recognition, glory and greatness to this free, yet priceless therapy otherwise considered to be nauseating. The whole world shall ever remain indebted to him for rendering this great humanitarian service." G.K.Thakkar

Manual for Urine Therapy is a modern day must have compendium for every possible use of urine to transform your health. His book is simple, informative, empowering and sprinkled with humor. Brother Sage is a gift to this community, as he translates ancient wisdom and healing practices, into practical and easy to use methods to integrate Shivambhu into your daily life. —Leila Sun (leilasun.com)

"Brother Sage has dug deep into the research and in his unique writing style and humor has birthed a new standard and approach to Urine Therapy. Readers will gain a rich understanding of the subject and find it easy to teach new folks the What, Why and How of reclaiming one's health with the UT Lifestyle."

"Every serious UT educator should have this Manual."
—Doc Mike Witort, Chicago, UT Therapist 21 years

"Brother Sage was responsible for the glee within me to burst out into laughter. I cannot forget his introduction to me, in that badly recorded song, " I am a pee drinking man." This was when I was a baby in Shivambhu, just started drinking my water.

Frankly speaking, I don't know how much of my healing was due to the Shivambhu, and how much to the Sangha. How much people like Brother Sage calling you a water family sister can truly empower the practice.

He inspired me, by his constant video posts of him drinking Shivambhu, without saying one word, to start the Facebook group, Shivambhu: Urine Therapy, India*(http://www.facebook.com/groups/2288913624455825)
An alternative therapy like Shivambhu can make life real lonesome, because all of your near and dear ones can make

You feel like you are crazy.

At such times, someone like Brother Sage stretches out his presence from thousands of miles across the planet to give you a virtual hug. I don't need to read his manuscript to know this is a fantastic book.

Thank you, Brother Sage, my water family.
—Manjushree Abhinav

Made in United States
Troutdale, OR
03/10/2024

18356980R00181